Advice for House Officers

Colin Johnson
MChir, FRCS

Senior Lecturer and Honorary Consultant Surgeon
University Surgical Unit, Southampton General Hospital
Southampton, UK

John Iredale
DM, MRCP

MRC Clinician Scientist and Honorary Senior Registrar
University Medicine, Southampton General Hospital
Southampton, UK

BEACONSFIELD PUBLISHERS LTD
Beaconsfield, Bucks, UK

This edition first published 1996

Previous edition:
(*Advice for House Surgeons*) published 1992, reprinted 1995

© C. D. Johnson and J. P. Iredale 1996

British Library Cataloguing in Publication Data
Johnson, C. D.
Advice for house officers
1. Hospitals – Medical staff – Handbooks, manuals, etc.
2. Medicine – Handbooks, manuals, etc.
I. Title II. Iredale, J. P.
610.6'952

ISBN 0–906584–43–4

Phototypeset by Gem Graphics, Trenance, Mawgan Porth, Cornwall in 10 on 12 point Times.
Printed and bound in Great Britain by The Bath Press, Somerset

Preface

This book is the distillation of many conversations with house physicians and house surgeons, some newly qualified who needed the advice contained in the following pages, and others nearing the end of their appointments who were able to advise us on the areas which had given them most difficulty. We hope it will serve as a 'survival kit' when you start these jobs, and also that it will help you to establish an open and friendly pattern of work for the years to come.

The information given here is necessarily generalised. Some details are specific to each hospital, and your own consultant may have different approaches in some areas – blank pages have been left at the end for you to make a note of local protocols and procedures. We are also conscious of the growing emphasis on education and counselling and have included sections on these topics, along with advice about contracts.

Read through the whole book before you start your house jobs and keep it handy for easy reference when awkward questions come up. Above all, we hope it will help you to get the most out of your pre-registration year, and enjoy it to the full.

Colin Johnson
John Iredale

Acknowledgements

We would like to express our thanks to Dr Mark Gaze, Dr Muir Gray, Mrs Margaret Johnston DipN, Mr Michael Pietroni and Dr Paul Reynolds. Each of them made time to read earlier or later drafts of the manuscript in detail, and we were pleased to be able to take their informed and thoughtful comments into account when preparing the final version.

CONTENTS

Asking for Advice and Assistance

You are not expected to know everything, just because you have passed Finals. If in doubt about how to handle any situation, ask for advice. Most experienced nurses will be very helpful, if you approach them in a sensible fashion. The nursing staff on your ward (particularly the Ward Manager) will have much practical experience which they will be pleased to share with you, if only you will ask. Seize any opportunity to befriend the hospital switchboard, senior porter and other ancillary staff. They may have the answer to your problem! Your SHO, registrar or senior registrar is there to help you learn how to manage patients.

Do not hesitate to ask for advice, day or night. Even if your registrar is off duty, it may be wise to ring him or her about a problem on the ward. Someone who knows the patient and the solution to the problem can usually deal with a question in two minutes over the telephone and save considerable time. Find out before the need arises how he or she would react to an out-of-hours request for advice. Most surgeons like to be informed at once if postoperative complications arise in their patients. Consultant physicians would usually wish to be informed of significant changes in the clinical condition of their patients, for example, transfer to ITU.

If you face a difficult situation, whether purely clinical or involving talking to an upset or angry patient or relative, always ask for advice beforehand. If you cannot get hold of a registrar, ring your consultant, who will probably be delighted to know that you have sufficient good sense not to exceed your capabilities. Two abilities characterise the house officer who is likely to learn most from his or her experience: (i) the ability to assess a situation and communicate accurately with senior staff, and (ii) the ability to recognise problems and seek advice before trouble arises.

It is conceivable, although unlikely, that you may reach a stage when you are so tired that you feel unable to think properly, or feel that you are becoming unreasonably clumsy or even a danger to your patients. If this should occur, do not blunder on (in a state of mistaken bravado) but speak to your SHO or Registrar, who will certainly be sympathetic. Your immediate senior in the oncall system should be in the hospital and immediately available to cover you for this type of crisis, as well as for the more likely event that you simply don't know how best to manage a patient. Do not hesitate to call for help in these circumstances. It may not be possible for you to withdraw immediately, but between you any remaining jobs can be reallocated to allow you to work safely and get some rest.

If you are asked to perform a procedure that you are not familiar with, always ask for assistance and supervision. We do not expect that anyone reading this book will be asked to undertake a new task unsupervised. In the unlikely event that you are put under pressure to do so, you must be resolute in requesting supervision – in the absence of such supervision you should not attempt a procedure that is beyond your competence. Do not yield to exhortations to 'just go ahead', or the peer group pressure of 'I taught myself', or the appeals to your pride of 'Well, Dr X has already done five'. If you are unhappy or unsure, always ask for help. That way you will always be safe and will be seen to have acted in the best interests of the patients, even if the result may have been temporary unpopularity with one of your colleagues. A good SHO/Registrar will never force you into an unsupported position.

As a pre-registration house officer you are completing your university training. You are not expected to take responsibilities and make decisions that cause you anxiety.

Remember: Ask before you act.
Always put the patient's best interests first.

Ward Rounds

Golden rules for ward rounds

- Anticipate your registrar's and your consultant's needs.
- Have available up-to-date results on all patients.
- Never sacrifice honesty to the desire to impress.
- *Never* make things up to cover your ignorance.
- Admit you don't know rather than hedge.
- Stay with the round.

Ward rounds are the times when decisions are made, management plans are confirmed and when unexpected problems are identified and dealt with. As a house officer you must be fully prepared for the round, so that complete and up-to-date information is available. You must record in the case notes the events of the ward round, and all decisions and plans made. You must write down all the things you will have to do in your own notebook, and you must make sure that all these decisions are carried out. In other words, you are the channel through which information reaches your senior colleagues, and you are the instrument which transforms their thoughts into action.

Build your routine around the ward rounds, as they all require some preparation and they all generate work.

Results

Results of patients should be available *in your hand or notebook* (i.e. *not* filed in the wrong place in the notes, which are on the trolley at the far end of the ward). You should be able to give accurate results as soon as they are asked for.

When asked for a result, give the numerical values, not 'Er . . . normal', or 'A bit raised'. Precision will impress; vagueness often suggests a cover for ignorance. However, never sacrifice honesty in the desire to impress. If you do not know – say so.

Results of blood tests *may* return spontaneously to the ward in time for the round. If they do not, find them in good time. Visit the laboratory or consult the computer system, to be sure you have the most recent results. It is impossible to plan fluid therapy, for example, on results that are over twenty-four hours old.

In order to have histology or radiology reports, you need to think ahead. Ring the relevant department two days before the ward round, to warn the pathologist or radiologist of your deadline. Allow time for the slides or images to be prepared and reported. You may not be able to have results at the last minute if there has been any delay in the routine processing.

During the round, avoid being distracted by your bleep, nurses or colleagues. Stay with the round. It is intensely irritating for your consultant if he or she asks the house officer a question, only to see a white coat tail disappearing round the door post to answer a bleep.

Consultant rounds (surgical)

Ward rounds with your consultant have several purposes. First, you need to show him or her new patients admitted for investigation or elective surgery. There may be patients who are recovering after treatment, and occasionally a patient with a persisting problem.

Your consultant may have another commitment to meet at a fixed time after the ward round. Begin the round by saying 'We have to go to A, B and C Wards as usual. In addition we have an outlying case on D Ward and a referral from the physician on E Ward.' Your consultant can then pace the round in the full knowledge of all the commitments.

New cases should be presented succinctly, with the patient's name, occupation, diagnosis and proposed operation stated first. This will help to remind the consultant about the patient, whom he has usually seen in the out-patient clinic. Mention any specific problems related to the operation, previous surgery, possible anaesthetic hazards (local or spinal anaesthesia may be indicated and the surgeon will want to know this in advance), and important social details. The patient may be the mother of the senior physician in the hospital, or she may live alone in an upstairs flat. Social factors such as these will influence the post-operative care of the patient and the need for convalescence. Make sure that you know the results of all investigations requested by the surgeon prior to admission, and have available all X-rays.

Sometimes it is irritatingly difficult to find the relevant X-ray in a thick X-ray folder. Prepare for this beforehand by separating the relevant films.

Second, you may have new emergency admissions which the consultant has not yet seen. These will be either diagnosed, operated on and recovered, or may still be undiagnosed. The first group should be presented succinctly. 'Mrs A.B. is 69 years old. She presented yesterday with small bowel obstruction. At laparotomy last night a band adhesion was divided, and the obstruction was relieved. No resection was necessary and she is making a good recovery. In the past she had a hysterectomy, and we think this was the cause of her adhesions.' Those who have been managed conservatively, or who are not yet diagnosed, require a fuller history and a description of the findings on examination. You must know the results of all investigations, as your consultant will be certain to ask.

Third, there may be patients who have been in hospital for some weeks, perhaps recovering from serious disease or surgical complications. Summarise the past events succinctly and note important recent developments. Don't assume your consultant remembers every detail from the last time the case was presented.

Consultant rounds (medical)

The approach to medical consultant rounds is broadly similar. Remind the consultant of the diagnosis and the reason for admission in those patients brought in for procedures. Summarise carefully the history, examination findings and results of previous tests for patients admitted for further investigations. Usually the majority of emergency admissions will have a diagnosis, e.g. 'This is Mrs C.D. who was admitted with chest pain on Tuesday. Her ECG demonstrated a clear inferior MI and she was given streptokinase. Subsequently she has experienced no complications.' – clear, precise and straightforward. For the more difficult emergency admissions (or routines) who have a diagnosis but are complicated in some way, simply relate the events and findings chronologically to date. If possible, avoid 'labelling' episodes with a diagnosis which may be erroneous. Let your senior make up his or her own mind. Similarly, if the patient does not have a clear diagnosis, relate the history as closely as possible to the way the patient described it when initially clerked. You have the advantage of taking the 'virgin' story before the patient puts emphasis on certain aspects, as a result of perceived interest by more senior members of the firm.

Finally, on either medical or surgical rounds, there will be some patients who have been seen on a previous ward round and who have had various investigations performed since then. It is your job to bring your chief up to date with the new results after a brief reminder of the problem. Make sure the X-ray films are on the ward, or else know where to find them. If the patient is having an investigation done at the time of the ward round, warn the radiologist that your consultant may come to look at the films at the end of the round. The radiologist can then keep the films handy, and won't send them off on a three-day tour of the hospital on their way 'back to the ward'.

Registrar rounds

These will take place at least once a day on the medical team, and on the surgical team possibly in both the mornings and evenings. Their purpose is to identify clinical problems, to decide the day's management tasks, and to review the day's results. It helps greatly if you have the facts assembled before the round starts. Ring the laboratory or check the computer to get important results before 5 p.m., when the laboratories close. It is very tedious to have to call in a biochemist at 5.35 p.m. to read out a result that has not been sent back to the ward. It seems to be always the sickest patient whose results are delayed or 'clotted'. Similarly, raid the X-ray Department for the day's films, so that your registrar can look at them.

Be aware of potential social problems which may affect the patient's recovery, rehabilitation and eventual discharge. Listen to what the nursing staff report about the social circumstances of each patient and make sure that relevant ancillary staff, e.g. physio and OT are involved early in the patient's care. A useful rule of thumb is to start thinking of a potential discharge date the day after admission. This rapidly disciplines you to think early in the patient's admission about any rehabilitation and social support that may be required.

Remember: Always look at patients' drug charts on the ward round, to identify those drugs which should be discontinued (e.g. opiates after the patient has survived the worst of the pain; antibiotics after 5–7 days).

On the Wards

Relationships with other staff

Your working life for the next few months will be based on your ward. It will be home from home for you, and it is in your interests to make friends with the people you work with – this makes life easier all round. Try to understand the problems of the nursing staff – their routine work, their shift system and why and where they are under-staffed. Many others will visit the ward – physiotherapists, occupational therapists, porters, cleaners, medical photographers, hospital managers and so on. Most have been there for some time, and will be there after you have gone. Remember that you have been sent there to work with them. They do not exist solely for your benefit. If you need help, or if something must be done, ask politely, and don't make blunt demands or give instructions. Nothing is more irritating for an experienced nurse or physiotherapist than to be told her job by someone who thinks they know better, but doesn't.

However, most of your colleagues of all disciplines will respond rapidly to the first signs that you can treat them as real people, especially if you can ask for and accept their advice where appropriate.

Ward work

In addition to clerking the patients and acting as a secretary for the ward rounds, as a house surgeon you will have to remember to obtain consent from every patient for theatre and other procedures, mark the site of the operation with an indelible pen where appropriate, and cross-match blood if necessary. Allow 24 hours of laboratory time for cross-matching – that is, send blood on Friday morning (or sooner) for a Monday morning list. On the medical ward your tasks will include organising the investigation of routine admissions and patients admitted for specialist tests, e.g. ERCP.

Endear yourself to the nurses by being tidy. Put notes back in the notes trolley after use. After taking blood or putting up drips, clear away the debris. Needles should go in the sharps box, not into someone's fingers. Do not try to resheathe needles after use – this increases the risk of stabbing yourself.

Do not expect the nursing staff to read your mind. Although it may sometimes seem that the staff nurse knows what you are going to do before you do yourself, you should still share with her all your innermost thoughts, at least as far as patient management is concerned. When you write up a drug or change an IV fluid regime, tell the nurse in charge. This will avoid arguments with nursing staff in front of the consultant: 'But I wrote that up yesterday!' . . . 'and we didn't know you had until after Pharmacy had closed!'

Nurses often have a very good 'feel' for the patients who are deteriorating and not quite right. Use their intuition to evaluate such patients carefully before physical signs appear.

When you wish to do a minor procedure, such as passing a urethral catheter, ask the nurse in charge if she can spare someone to help you. Be prepared to list the items you will require on the trolley, and try not to forget anything. You will rarely feel more foolish than when you are left alone behind curtains with a half-catheterised patient, waiting for a nurse who doesn't know the ward to find and bring you a catheter bag or syringe.

Referrals

- Referrals to the firm should be seen the same day.
- Don't forget about the referral card once it has gone into your pocket.

Referrals from other firms should be seen by the registrar the same day. This is important, as it demonstrates that your firm provides a good service to your colleagues, and encourages a flow of patients in both directions. Inform your consultant of referrals as soon as possible, and at the latest at the *start* of the next ward round. It can be infuriating for your consultant to get to the end of the round and suddenly to be faced with three patients to go and see, instead of a relaxing chat with Sister over a cup of coffee.

Case notes

Case notes are used for many purposes:
1) To ensure planning and continuity of care.
2) For communication between doctors and other staff.
3) To enable another doctor to assume care of the patient at any time.

4) To provide documentary evidence of course and management.
5) To allow evaluation of clinical care.
6) They are a record of data for research and education.
7) To protect the legal interests of (i) patient, (ii) staff and
   (iii) hospital.

It is your responsibility to maintain the clinical records. Always record clearly the date and time of each entry. When patients are admitted to hospital you must clerk them in and record your findings in the notes. State whether it is an emergency or an elective admission, and record clearly the name of the consultant with responsibility for the patient. Results of any investigations should be entered in the notes in red ink to make them more obvious (although some hospitals discourage this, because red reproduces poorly on microfilm). It will help you think clearly about your findings on history and examination if you formulate and record a differential diagnosis. This is especially useful when problems arise; and with emergency admissions it is a routine you should go through *before* contacting a senior colleague, wherever possible.

Your responsibilities do not stop at the time of operation or after initial medical management. It is important to make a record of every patient's progress, and to record in the notes the findings and diagnosis made by the consultant, any change in management, and finally the date of discharge.

The case notes are legal documents and their maintenance is your responsibility. Remember that patients have a right of access to their notes and do not write derogatory comments or make unjustifiable accusations. This is offensive and may make difficulties for you later. For example, don't write: 'Admitted drunk', but do record the evidence: 'Smelling of whisky, unable to stand, and abusive'.

Make an entry in the case notes at least every day, more often if the clinical condition is changing. This is important not only medico-legally, but also to convey up-to-date information to those of your colleagues who may provide night-time cover. Sign every entry, and make sure the patient's name is written on every sheet – notes can fall apart! Record every manipulation of the patient (catheter inserted, drip down, etc.). Even if your hospital uses separate operation sheets, record the name of any operations or procedures in red in its chronological place in the patient's notes. Write histology and cytology reports in the notes in red when they become available. You may be asked to write up the operation note, although many surgeons prefer to do this themselves. Describe the incision, findings (normal and abnormal), and the results of intra-operative investigations such as cholangiograms and frozen sections. Record the procedure carried out, and any intra-operative difficulties (be honest!). Note the presence of any drains and catheters, and finally note the method of wound closure and suture material used. Postoperative instructions should be written on the operation note. A diagram of the findings or of the procedure is often helpful.

If you speak to a patient or relatives about the diagnosis, particularly of cancer or other incurable illness, record exactly what you have said in the notes. It is important for successive doctors to know exactly what has been said.

Remember:
• Date every entry.
• Sign each entry legibly.
• If the patient belongs to another team, write your bleep number, grade and consultant after your entry in the notes.

Discharges

The discharge form may serve two purposes:
1) It tells the GP about the inpatient treatment and potential problems.
2) It records information of work done for the hospital accounting system.

You need to record:
• Dates of admission and discharge.
• Ward, and consultant in charge.
• Diagnosis.
• All relevant investigations performed and their results (e.g. blood tests, CT scans).
• All procedures done – e.g. colonoscopy and biopsy; endoscopic polypectomy (not just 'polypectomy'); or cholecystectomy and exploration of common bile duct (not just 'operation for gallstones').
• Patient's condition at discharge (e.g. 'Cardiac failure controlled on diuretics', or 'The surgical wound has healed, sutures to be removed').
• Information given to patients and relatives.

- Arrangements for immediate care (e.g. for the district nurse to call).
- Arrangements for outpatient follow-up.
- Medication on discharge.
- Any special request to GP for follow-up or adjustment of medication.

All hospitals now record details of inpatient treatment at the time of discharge from hospital. This information is used to calculate the workload of your unit and thus to allocate the appropriate budget. It is clearly essential that these forms (currently HMR1) are completed fully and clearly, so that coding clerks can give correct codes for all procedures carried out. You should complete these forms fully, on the day the patient is discharged. When a patient leaves hospital, inform his general practitioner. The most convenient and effective way to do this is to give the patient a discharge letter which he takes to his doctor's surgery during the week after discharge from hospital. Record on this form the diagnosis and brief details of inpatient treatment; tell the general practitioner of any changes in long-term medication; and ask the patient to be sure to deliver the letter to the surgery or give it to his doctor when he next visits.

If any problems are likely to arise, for example if the patient has a discharging wound, or controlled cardiac failure, it is courteous to telephone and speak directly to the general practitioner. Alternatively, you can send a fax to the GP's surgery.

If the patient requires a district nurse to visit, the nursing staff on the ward will usually arrange this directly.

It is even more important to inform the patient's general practitioner if the patient dies in hospital. You should do this at the latest by 9 a.m. on the next normal working day.

Remember: The main purpose of contacting the GP is to provide warning of any potential problems, whether these relate to patient management or bereaved relatives.

What to Carry in Your Pockets

An efficient house officer will strike the right balance between carrying sufficient equipment and reference material to do the job effectively, and being so overburdened with bits and pieces that it is impossible to find the right thing at the right time.

Things to have with you

The most important tasks of a house officer are to record information, and to carry out instructions of senior colleagues. You should always start the day with three pens. One will run out, you will lose one, and you will still have one to write with. Varied colours are less important, and although a red pen may be useful for highlighting important results it is better to write the result in black or blue and circle it in red if you wish, to ensure that the original record can be microfilmed or photocopied accurately.

You will need a notebook. A looseleaf ringbinder can be useful, if you are prepared to use a separate page for each patient and keep each page up to date. You will need to take the time to look through all the pages at the beginning and end of each day. It may be more practical to have a simple notebook into which you write all the things that need to be done, and cross them off as they are completed. You should check your notebook before going off duty and make sure that all essential tasks have been completed, or handed over to the on-call house officer.

Before going off duty, make a list of tasks for the next day. In the morning, write down everything which arises from the morning ward round and then, before you start working on all of these tasks, put them in order of priority. If you begin each new day on a new page in your notebook you will know where you are, and you will have all your work in one place.

Most hospitals use computerised patient identification systems which print the patient's name and address, general practitioner, hospital number and other details onto a sticky label. Acquire a supply of blank labels and keep some in your pocket at all times. These are useful for recording telephone messages about patients (for example biochemistry results) when you do not have immediate access to their notes. Always write the patient's name and the time and date on each label as you record the information. It is then a simple matter to transfer this to the hospital notes without having to copy everything out.

The only book you need to carry with you is a British National Formulary (BNF). The BNF lists all prescribed drugs, and will help you to identify the patient's medication. This may be known to the patient by one of a number of trade names, or you may only be able to get a description ('the little white pills for my heart, Doctor'). If you check their identity immediately, the patient's memory may be jogged and you can confirm the correct name of the tablets. Most wards will have a BNF on their drug trolley, but you may be clerking the patient in an unfamiliar ward or in the accident department, and it is more efficient to carry your own copy.

Always carry a tourniquet.

Personal needs

The life of a house officer is unpredictable and you may work for several hours without interruption when a take night is busy. Under these circumstances it may be difficult to find time for your own needs. When called during the night you may leave essential supplies in your room. The list of possible standbys could be overwhelming. The following suggestions highlight some important items to keep in your white coat:

Loose change to purchase food/drink in the night.

A chocolate bar or other emergency food supply.

Any small personal items whose ready availability may be important to you.

Two or three spare doses of any medication you take regularly.

If you deal with any paediatric patients, a small toy, rattle or fluffy object may help to divert attention while you examine a child.

The unpredictable demands of allergic or infective rhinitis can be met by paper towels or tissues from the ward.

Books

There is no need to carry large volumes of printed material with you. The BNF is essential, and as already mentioned, you should have your own notebook. Other books (see suggested reading at the end of this book) are best kept for handy reference in places where you are likely to use them, such as the doctors' office on the ward. One exception might be this book, which you may wish to keep handy for immediate reference. Write down, in the pages provided at the back, all the frequently used telephone numbers you require, and your local protocols for emergency treatment of some common conditions.

Useful bits of equipment

Stethoscope
Tourniquet
A pen torch
Your own tube of lubricating jelly and a spare glove
A couple of tongue depressors
A roll of adhesive tape.
Ophthalmoscope (on a medical job)
A small patella hammer

All of these items are useful during clinical examination, and it is more convenient to carry your own than to search for them, especially on an unfamiliar ward. Carry a roll of tape to apply immediate reinforcement to insecure IV lines or partly-removed dressings.

Look at the pockets of the other trainees on your firm and ask yourself whether you are carrying around more material than they are, and if so, whether you need it all.

What to avoid

There is little point in carrying around items that are better kept in the ward office. Textbooks are heavy and of little help in face-to-face contact. You are better to have these available where you sit to write the notes, so that you can check things as you think about them.

Tape measures are cumbersome and get tangled up with everything else. It is better to have a 15cm ruler in your pocket. If a tape measure is essential because of the nature of the patients you see, get one which retracts into its own plastic case.

An ophthalmoscope is redundant on most surgical wards. You may find one useful doing a medical job, but it is only worth carrying one if you are trained and confident in its use.

Sphygmomanometry is best done using fixed equipment, which you will often find attached to the wall in Casualty cubicles, Outpatient consulting rooms and pre-clerking areas. Handy pocket sphygmomanometers are neither handy nor do they fit in your pocket, and it is probably best to use the ward equipment.

Routine Medical Admissions

Routine medical admissions fall into two groups. A relatively large number of patients are admitted as day cases or overnight cases for procedures. The nature of the procedures and your role in assessing these patients will very much depend upon the firm that you work with. The other routine admissions, which are usually smaller in number, are those patients admitted for a programme of investigations. Both groups of patients must be clerked on the day of admission.

The secret to sorting out routine admissions painlessly is to plan your day carefully. Often patients arrive first thing in the morning for a procedure later that day. It is therefore vital that you prioritise obtaining the relevant tests. Ensure that the results of tests already done are on the ward in advance of the patient's arrival. Get the day's results back in time before the patient goes down to X-ray, endoscopy, etc.

Remember: Written consent will be required for all procedures listed below. You should therefore be aware of what is involved in each procedure, its risk, and any possible complications that might be expected. Always clearly warn patients of any likely discomfort they may expect.

The following list covers the common tests for which patients are admitted as routines and the blood tests which are usually required.

- *Renal biopsy.* These patients require an IVP. This has to be very up-to-date and is often performed on the day before admission. The films must be available to go down with the patient. Usually blood and urine are collected for the biochemical indices of renal function, such as creatinine clearance. Make sure you have the results of a full blood count and clotting screen and that a sample has gone to Blood Transfusion to be grouped and saved. In addition, check an MSU to ensure that there is no bacterial growth in the urine. Lastly, before the patient leaves the ward, insert an IV cannula.
- *Cardiac catheters.* These patients may have been relatively extensively investigated in Outpatients and therefore already have up-to-date blood tests. However, cardiologists frequently use the opportunity of admission to obtain up-to-date fasting plasma

15

specimens for lipid and cholesterol measurement. Check the policy in your hospital. At a minimum, the patients should have their full blood count and clotting documented and blood should be grouped and saved. Make sure there is a current PA and left lateral chest X-ray and ECG, and place an IV cannula.

- *Bronchoscopy.* Patients admitted for bronchoscopy often have a degree of respiratory failure. Always document the blood gases on the day of admission. In addition all patients require PA and lateral chest films, pulmonary function tests and an ECG. Make sure these are available to go with the patient.
- *Liver biopsy.* Patients with liver disease frequently have deranged clotting, and this may lead to the procedure being cancelled. Check the patient's clotting and platelet counts on the day of the procedure, and if either are deranged discuss the case with the doctor performing the procedure. In addition send blood to be grouped and saved, and insert an IV cannula. Injection of varices is like liver biopsy: the clotting and platelet count should be documented. Send blood to be grouped and saved, and site an IV cannula.
- *ERCP.* The patient's clotting and platelets should be checked. Again, the persons performing the procedure should be made aware of derangements in clotting time or platelet count. An IV cannula is also required as routine, usually in the right hand or arm.

Remember: Jaundiced patients may have vitamin K deficient coagulopathy, and this should be corrected before any procedure.

There are some routine medical investigations for which a doctor is required to be present and this role may fall to the house officer. Two examples of this are the (cardiology) exercise tolerance test and the (endocrine) insulin stress test. The nature of these tests is that they stress the patient – you should therefore familiarise yourself with the local protocol used and determine precisely what your role is. Ask your registrar if you have doubts or are unclear about anything. The technical staff involved in these tests will usually be extremely helpful and supportive. Familiarise yourself with the changes in the patient's vital signs as well as the ECG changes that may occur during stress testing, so that you know when to intervene and terminate the investigation.

Finally, there are patients who are admitted for investigation because in some way they are not straightforward. These have usually been seen in the clinic by the registrar or consultant and, by definition, are difficult and complex cases. Although they may take some time to clerk, often with an extensive past medical history, they may be highly educational. A vital part of this is to document carefully what is present in the patient's case notes, especially the results of pertinent previous tests. Indeed, if you can construct a proper differential diagnosis and problem list, you may well cast light on the case or pick up a diagnosis that has been missed by your consultant or registrar. This is an excellent way to make a memorable good impression – but don't overdo it. Let the consultant choose the right diagnosis from your list of suggestions.

Preoperative Investigation and Administration

All patients must be seen by a house surgeon and clerked and examined on the day of admission. This is *essential*. How would you feel if you were a patient, and no one came to see you on your first day in hospital? How would you feel if a patient of yours died in the night, and you had not clerked her?

In addition to clerking the patients, you must also request appropriate investigations and find the results of recent tests if they have been done. In particular, you must ensure that all investigations requested at the last outpatient visit have been done and that the results are available. Investigations which have a direct bearing on the decision to operate are particularly important. For example, your consultant may well wish to see ultrasound scans which demonstrate gallstones before cholecystectomy, or barium enema films before a colonic resection.

When patients are admitted to hospital on the day before surgery, you will improve the chances of getting the results that day if you take blood to the lab yourself before midday. Hospital porters may sometimes be unreliable and slow, because they may not appreciate the urgency of the samples they are handling. If you put in a personal appearance in the laboratory, and exchange a few words with the technical staff, this can have a remarkable effect on the proportion of results which come back to you before 5 p.m.!

Day cases

You may be required to clerk patients who are admitted to the ward for day case surgery under local or general anaesthesia. For minor operations under local anaesthesia, and for procedures such as check cystoscopy, you need only do a brief clerking. Five minutes should be enough to do that. Spend another five minutes to explain the procedure and to obtain consent. Establish the patient's identity and the nature of his complaint. Note any other medical condition and any drug allergies. Ask specifically about any changes since previous general anaesthetics. Briefly examine the relevant parts (including the cardiorespiratory system for all general anaesthetic cases).

Obtain consent from all patients, even if they will be conscious for the procedure. The operating theatre staff will insist on this detail.

General anaesthetic cases

Your hospital may have a policy for minimum preoperative investigations. Find out from the Anaesthetic Department what they will require. As a rule of thumb, you will need the following minimum investigations:

Over 40 years, full blood count.
Over 50 years, full blood count + electrocardiogram (ECG).
Over 60 years, full blood count + plasma urea and electrolytes (U&E) + chest X-ray + ECG.

Additional investigations will be required for specific indications. Younger patients with a history of cardiorespiratory disease will require appropriate investigations. Your anaesthetist will advise you on which patients should have respiratory function tests such as forced respiratory volumes and peak flows.

In patients with a high alcohol intake, a prothrombin time is more important than liver enzymes. The patient may need vitamin K pre-operatively. Anyone with a history of jaundice should be tested for hepatitis B antigen and hepatitis C antibodies. All Asian patients should have a chest X-ray, to exclude tuberculosis. Afro-Caribbean patients need to have a sickle test before any general anaesthetic. This can be done immediately on the sample taken for haemoglobin estimation. Patients with rheumatoid arthritis will need an X-ray of the cervical spine for the benefit of the anaesthetist.

All homosexuals, drug addicts, haemophiliacs, and those who have had large blood transfusions, or transfusions in Central Africa, are at risk of carrying both HIV and hepatitis B. It is rare for patients to take exception to questions on these subjects if the purpose is made clear. Patients with a history of potential exposure should be tested for evidence of infection with these agents only after they have given informed consent. Because of the implications – not just of a positive result but even the fact of having had an HIV test – all patients should be offered proper counselling prior to an HIV test being done. A patient who is at high risk of infection and refuses to give consent for a blood test should be treated as if he or she were infected. Your hospital will have special procedures for dealing with inoculation risk patients in the operating theatre. (See also pages 60–1.)

Long-term drug therapy

- Always inform anaesthetists of long-term therapy.
- Very few drugs need to be stopped before surgery.
- Anticoagulants pose special problems.
- Oral contraceptives, lithium, some antidepressants should be stopped three to four weeks before surgery.
- Oral hypoglycaemics should be stopped on the day of surgery.
- Most drugs can be given on the day of operation.
- Some drugs *must* be continued in the preoperative period: anticonvulsants, clonidine and possibly adrenocorticosteroids.

If possible, confirm current therapy with the GP, and examine the patient's medicine bottles.

Patients who are on long-term medication before they come into hospital may require adjustments in their therapy in relation to the anaesthetic. In addition, some long-term treatments will require a different anaesthetic technique. Inform the anaesthetist of any such medication. In particular, discuss the management of diabetic patients and those who are taking antihypertensive drugs or steroids.

Patients for elective surgery should discontinue monoamine oxidase inhibitors two weeks before operation, and the oral contraceptive should be discontinued for four weeks. It may be necessary to delay surgery to achieve this. Patients taking warfarin may have to be converted to heparin for the period of the operation, because this allows easier reversal of the anticoagulation if haemorrhage occurs. All anticoagulated patients require daily monitoring of the degree of anticoagulation. This should be done in consultation with the Haematology Department. Patients on heparin are monitored with activated partial thromboplastin times, and those on warfarin need prothrombin times, but many local variations on these groups of tests exist.

Remember: If a patient needs a drug before he comes into hospital, he probably needs it before (and after) the operation.

Cross-matching

Find out if your blood bank operates a policy for cross-matching blood for elective surgery. Try to keep to these guidelines, but check with your registrar or consultant. Order blood in good time to enable the lab to do the cross-match in normal working hours, before the start of the list. You will need to order blood at least 24 hours in advance for all gastrointestinal resections, arterial cases, and open urological and orthopaedic cases. Ideally, provide more leeway, to allow for difficult cross-matching of patients with unusual antibodies.

Cross-matched blood for surgical cases is usually stored in a refrigerator in or close to the operating theatre. You can check that the blood is available for theatre by looking in this refrigerator.

Blood is a scarce resource and should be used efficiently. Your blood bank may provide packed cells and plasma expanders, which are adequate in most elective situations.

Recently-transfused blood is not an efficient oxygen transporter. Find out from your anaesthetist whether an anaemic patient should be transfused preoperatively (more than 48 hours is ideal) or during the operation.

On the day before elective cases, check that the blood has been cross-matched and is available. Tell the blood bank if the operation is postponed or cancelled, or if the patient is not going to use the blood. Unused blood is recalled after 48 hours to be cross-matched for other patients.

Anticoagulation

Heparinising a patient is a dangerous procedure and should be monitored closely. Heparin requirements change rapidly, and should be monitored twice daily at first with kaolin cephalin times (KCT) or activated partial thromboplastin times (APT). The results are usually expressed as a ratio to a control value. You can reduce the element of guesswork in setting the dose by using the following protocol (Fennerty et al., BMJ, **292**, 579–80, 1986):

Loading dose: 5000 units over 5 minutes.

Infusion: Start at 1400 units/hour, that is 8400 units in 100 ml over 6 hours. Then adjust the dose according to the ratio of KCT to control values, using the following table (overleaf).

Ratio	Change in heparin infusion rate
Greater than 5	Reduce by 500 u/h
4.1–5	Reduce by 300 u/h
3.1–4	Reduce by 100 u/h
2.6–3	Reduce by 50 u/h
1.5–2.5	No change
1.2–1.4	Increase by 200 u/h
Less than 1.2	Increase by 400 u/h

Wait 10 hours before the next estimation of KCT unless the ratio is greater than 5, in which case more frequent estimation is advisable.

Prophylactic antibiotics

Most surgeons have a clearly defined policy for prophylactic anti-biotics. Find out your chief's requirements as soon as possible. Broadly speaking, during the operation and for the following 12 to 24 hours, there should be an adequate concentration of antibiotic in the plasma to prevent implanted organisms infecting the wound. Upper gastrointestinal surgery is covered by antibiotics active against Gram-negative bacilli. A second-generation cephalosporin is usually given. Colorectal surgery requires an agent active against anaerobes, such as metronidazole, in addition to the cephalosporin. Urological procedures are also covered by an agent active against Gram-negative bacilli – a broad spectrum penicillin or a cephalosporin would be useful. In vascular and orthopaedic surgery, skin organisms may contaminate the implant, so these patients require an agent with proven activity against staphylococci. When writing up prophylactic antibiotics always specify the number of doses to be given (1–3 is usually sufficient), and mark the chart appropriately to discontinue after this time. This will avoid inappropriate long-term treatment.

Prophylaxis against deep vein thrombosis (DVT)

Most surgeons hold strong views on this subject and you should find out as soon as possible what policy your consultant wishes you to follow. You might ask on your first ward round, 'Do you wish all patients for laparotomy to have subcutaneous heparin, or only "high-risk" cases?' You should know that high-risk cases include patients over 40, the obese, smokers, those with malignant disease or undergo-ing pelvic operations, and those with a history of DVT. The nurse in charge of the ward will tell you whether or not your consultant likes all patients to wear elastic anti-embolism stockings.

Patients taking the oral contraceptive or oestrogen-based hormone replacement therapy should have this discontinued one month before surgery. If this is not possible, prophylactic measures against DVT should be used for *any* operation in these patients.

When you start your medical job, you will also be looking after patients at risk of DVT, for example, after myocardial infarction. Remember this and discuss with your registrar or consultant which patients merit anti-DVT prophylaxis on the medical ward.

Miscellaneous tips

- *Thyroid.* When you admit a patient for thyroid surgery, make sure that the results of any recent investigations are available. In particular try to find the serum thyroxine results, thyroid antibody tests, and scans. If the patient has not had an indirect laryngoscopy, arrange for this to be done. This is to check that both vocal cords are moving before the laryngeal nerves are exposed at operation. Postoperatively, check for stridor and neck swelling and ask the patient about tingling, check for signs of tetany, and send blood for a serum calcium in case the parathyroid glands have been destroyed.
- *Arterial.* When clerking arterial cases, listen for any bruits in the carotid and femoral pulses. If the patient has come in for surgery, it is essential to find the films of any arteriograms. Always measure the arterial pressures in the foot pulses using a Doppler probe. It saves time on the ward round if you write the pressures on the patient at the site of the pulse as well as writing them in the notes.
- *Intensive care.* Patients who are about to have really major surgery, such as oesophagectomy or aortic reconstruction, will go to the Intensive Care Unit postoperatively. Book a bed on ITU as soon as possible. Many ITUs welcome a preoperative visit from the patient, who can then be forewarned about some of the routines and meet the nurses. This is very reassuring to the patient, who will undoubtedly be scared stiff at the thought of the operation and the postoperative care. Speak to the ITU team before sending the patient down!

Remember: Inform the surgeon and anaesthetist of any potential problems or cancellations. Never agree to change the list without the consent of the surgeon and anaesthetist.

Pre-admission Clinics

Many patients who are to be admitted for routine procedures are asked to attend pre-admission clinics. In some hospitals these are known as pre-clerking clinics. The purpose of this type of clinic is to screen the patient for conditions which will affect their management in hospital, and to ensure that all necessary investigations have been completed before the procedure. This approach enables patients to be admitted on the day of operation, rather than the day before, thereby saving occupation of a hospital bed and shortening their stay.

You may well be required to clerk patients in the pre-admission clinic. If you remember the function of this clinic, you will save yourself time and contribute to the smooth running of the firm. For example, when clerking a fit young patient before a hernia repair, it is rarely necessary to obtain a detailed family history, or go through an exhaustive list of questions enquiring after symptoms in every system. The following questions *are* important:

What is the presenting complaint?
What is the planned procedure?
Are there any symptoms suggesting complications?

Cardiorespiratory system
Do you suffer from shortness of breath?
Have you had any chest pain?
Have you ever been treated for high blood pressure?
Have you ever had a heart attack?

General questions
Are you taking any medication?
Are you on any long-term treatment? (Specifically ask about oral contraceptives, insulin, warfarin, anti-depressants, 'heart pills' and anti-hypertensives.)
Do you have any allergies?

Social circumstances

It is particularly important when day case surgery or early discharge is intended, to establish that the patient will be adequately cared for

24

during the immediate recovery period. Record in the notes what arrangements the patient has made for care at home during the first forty-eight hours after discharge.

Does the patient live alone?
Does he or she live in a flat or house with stairs?
Is there easy access to bathing and toilet facilities?
Is there a telephone (to summon emergency help if necessary)?

For day cases it is imperative that the patient should be accompanied on the journey home, and should not drive home from the hospital. After a general anaesthetic, patients should be supervised by a responsible person for twenty-four hours.

What to do about a problem

If you discover any unexpected medical condition, medication, or social circumstance which may prevent the planned procedure being carried out, inform the anaesthetist and the surgeon. **Make plans to deal with the necessary change in any operating list.** One of the great advantages of a pre-admission clinic is that any problems are detected several days before the planned list. This will enable a substitute patient to be called to fill the gap if your patient is cancelled. Appropriate decisions can be made about discontinuation of medication before a general anaesthetic. Do not waste these opportunities by failing to communicate with your senior colleagues.

If a patient fails to attend for a pre-clerking appointment, it is likely that they will not attend for the operation. Ensure that an attempt is made to contact the patient to determine why they have not attended, and if necessary arrange for another patient to be sent for to cover the gap.

Informed Consent

It is the responsibility of the surgeon or physician carrying out a procedure to make sure that the patient has given fully informed consent to that procedure. Ideally the operator will obtain this consent personally, but in many instances the duty will be delegated to the house officer. It is a legal requirement that a patient should give informed consent before submitting to any procedure, and it can be argued in law that if the consent was not properly informed then it is invalid.

If you are obtaining consent for operation from a patient, make sure that you understand what the procedure involves and what the likely outcomes might be. You should mention any possible complications which might be life-threatening or have a permanent adverse effect on the patient's quality of life, for example an anastomotic leakage or recurrent laryngeal nerve injury during thyroid procedures. In British law, complications which are very unlikely need not be specifically mentioned – for example, it is not negligent to omit mention of fatal pulmonary embolus after cholecystectomy – but in contrast it could be held negligent to avoid any discussion of bile duct injury in that operation.

If you have any doubts about what is appropriate, make sure you check with a senior colleague what should be said, and ideally bring the surgeon/physician and the patient together and listen to their conversation.

If a patient refuses to give consent, inform the surgeon as soon as possible. Appropriate consent forms are available for patients who refuse blood transfusions. The operating surgeon and anaesthetist *must* be made aware of these patients before the start of the list.

Consent for minors should be obtained from a parent or legal guardian. In extreme circumstances (e.g. where the patient is unconscious) consent should be obtained from the next of kin. If the next of kin is unknown or not available, report this at once to your registrar, who will ensure that the necessary decisions are taken.

Specific areas of consent require special mention

- *Stoma formation.* Establish before you talk to the patient whether the operation will involve the creation of a stoma. If this is possible but not certain, try to find out the degree of likelihood from the surgeon involved. You can then deal with this question appropriately. Make sure you know whether any stoma will be temporary or permanent, and find out if possible what type of stoma will be created (ileostomy or colostomy), in order to warn the patient about potential problems such as high fluid output after ileostomy.

- *Nephrectomy.* Make sure that the patient understands that the removal of one kidney makes the other kidney especially 'valuable'. They should be warned that any injury in the area of the remaining kidney could lead to renal failure, and their medical attendants should be informed of the previous nephrectomy. You should make sure that the opposite kidney has been shown to have normal function before a nephrectomy.

- *Impotence and sexual function.* Operations in the pelvis, particularly those involving removal of the rectum or bladder, may damage the pelvic nerves and lead to impotence or impairment of sexual function. The possibility of this should be discussed with the patient, irrespective of his or her age; if you are unsure of the likely effects of the operation, ask the surgeon to do this.

- *Sterilisation.* Anyone having a sterilisation should understand that the procedure is normally irreversible, but that there is a very small risk of failure.

- *Endoscopy.* For routine upper and lower GI endoscopy the likelihood of serious complications following the procedure is very small, provided that the patients have been fasted for an appropriate time and have taken any relevant bowel preparation. Failure to comply with preparatory instructions can make the procedure hazardous, and should always be checked before consent is obtained. Patients going for ERCP should be warned that the procedure may produce discomfort and the small risk of post-sphincterotomy bleeding, and the nature of stenting and other biliary manipulation should be explained clearly. All ERCP procedures are associated with a small risk of pancreatitis. For patients undergoing bronchoscopic examination, the small risk of pneumothorax after transbronchial biopsy should be discussed – don't forget to arrange a post-examination chest X-ray in such patients.

- *Cardiac catheters.* When obtaining consent, the patient should be warned of the small possibility of ischaemic damage occurring during the procedure. If the patient is undergoing angioplasty, then the possibility of coronary artery damage should be mentioned. In both cases patients must understand that urgent bypass surgery may be required.
- *Liver biopsy/Renal biopsy.* Both of these procedures are very safe and are now often performed under ultrasound guidance. When consent is obtained, the patient should be warned that there can be pain (often described as being 'like a dull kick') after the procedure. In addition there is the small but finite risk of haemorrhage from the biopsy site, and in the case of the liver, of biliary peritonitis.

Laparoscopic surgery

Minimally invasive surgery has become widespread in the last few years, but patients should be aware that it is occasionally necessary to convert to an open procedure. In most cases the risk of this is 5 per cent or less and can be put to the patient as 'about a one in 20 chance'.

Tubes and drains

Indicate if possible to the patient the likely siting of any catheters, drainage tubes and nasogastric tubes. This is particularly important if the operation may involve a colostomy, because the patient will wish to know as soon as he or she has recovered whether a colostomy has been necessary, and may confuse a drainage tube with a colostomy appliance. It is also less likely to generate unnecessary anxiety if the patient is expecting to have a drainage tube, should one be necessary.

Planned admissions to intensive care and high dependency

Many major procedures require postoperative care in the ITU or HDU. If this seems likely it should be explained to the patient beforehand. If possible, a visit to the ITU or the HDU should be arranged so that the patient can become familiar with these very strange surroundings. The unit staff will show the patient where they will be nursed, and will explain the bewildering array of equipment around the bed. Such a visit should be arranged in advance with the nurse in charge of the unit.

Anticipate postoperative care and discharge

The patient should be aware of the plans made for his or her post-operative management and the likely date of discharge from hospital. Many patients are still surprised to be told that they can leave hospital the day after cholecystectomy. Forewarned is forearmed, and forward planning will enable you to keep control of your bed occupancy. Particular areas of postoperative management involve those cases which will require dressings after discharge from hospital, for example laying open of a fistula in ano, or open treatment of a pilonidal sinus. If the surgeon wishes the patient to wear a stocking for a prolonged period after surgery for varicose veins, this should be explained before the operation.

Request Cards and Referrals

Fill in all forms fully and clearly. Remember that if you use sticky labels for the patient's details, you will need to attach one to all copies of multiple copy forms (or else write the details by hand!).

Follow the laboratory's instructions for filling in the forms. This will help the efficient handling of your requests and may get your results back on time. For example, if the form requests only one tick on a row of boxes, then you have to write a separate request for more than one test. Remember that it will be quicker to do this than to try and retrieve a lost specimen or have an extra test done out of hours.

Give clear reasons for the request in the space marked 'Clinical Details'. State the question you want answered, which should help the pathologist or radiologist to focus on the problem. This way your firm will obtain the maximum of valuable information from the pathologist or radiologist. If it doesn't make sense to you, ask your registrar 'Why?' before you have to answer the same question from an equally puzzled laboratory or radiology department.

Emergency Admissions

The golden rule is to do what the registrar tells you, because he or she is directly involved in all emergency admissions and takes responsibility for their management.

All referrals direct from general practitioners should be accepted. This applies even to cases which you may think are not related to your speciality. You can then sort them out when they have arrived. Be polite to the general practitioner – who is usually doing his or her best under difficult circumstances. You will see the force of this argument much more clearly when you are fully registered, and perhaps from the other side of the fence if you work in general practice.

To get a flavour of the family doctor's problems, imagine the following exercise. Ring another hospital while three friends are watching you and waiting impatiently to go off duty. Ask to speak to the Urology house officer. The switchboard will then erroneously connect you to the Neurology SHO and then to the medical house officer. After you have explained the details of your case to each of these in turn, you will wait for five minutes as you hold on a dead line while the switchboard loses your call. Finally you will have to write a letter to the urologist and send it via the Emergency Bed Service, before you go off with your colleagues to moan about hospital switchboards, arrogant SHOs and rude house officers (in the other hospital, of course). The general practitioner has to face this every day, ringing from the home of a patient and surrounded by anxious relatives. He or she then has to arrange an ambulance to bring the patient to hospital. Have some sympathy with their problems.

When you accept an emergency referral, tell the Casualty reception and the ward nurse, so that old notes can be searched for and preparations made to receive the patient.

Remember to ask the referring doctor for the patient's hospital number so that Casualty or the ward clerk can get out the old notes. It is often useful to note the GP's name and telephone number, so that you can check any points which may need clarification after the patient has arrived. Ask the GP to send all current medication to the hospital with the patient.

You may also be asked to deal with referrals from casualty officers in the hospital. Such referrals fall into two groups. There are those cases which the casualty officer feels need admission. Admit these patients to hospital as efficiently as possible. Other patients may be referred to the firm for an opinion as to whether they need admission. Pass these directly on to your registrar. It is not your place as a house officer to send patients home from Casualty.

Surgical emergencies

When you deal with emergency surgical admissions, organisation is essential. You must establish appropriate priorities. For example, it would be wrong to spend time with a middle-aged man who has an irreducible hernia, before you deal with a child who has had severe abdominal pain and vomiting for two days. Be guided by your registrar if you have to make such choices. Try to see the life-threatening condition first, and as efficiently as possible.

It is often helpful to make an initial immediate assessment. If it is clear that the patient will require intravenous fluids and an operation, set up a drip, take blood and arrange for an ECG *before* spending time on a full history and examination. That way, treatment has started and the blood results will be available by the time you have finished your clerking.

Medical emergencies

Much of your time as a medical house officer will be spent clerking medical emergencies. This chapter is not a substitute for a textbook. Get a good pocket-sized text on medical emergencies and keep it handy. A useful book is: *Medical Emergencies – Diagnosis and Management* by Robinson and Stott.

Hospitals differ in their policies for arranging emergency admissions; you may receive the GP calls directly, whereas in some hospitals they are put through to your SHO or registrar or the Bed Bureau, who will arrange admission wherever there is a free bed. If you are in charge of taking the GP calls, remember that however tired and fed up you feel, the general practitioner is probably in the same state and has probably been hanging on the telephone for some considerable time. Always be polite and courteous. Always accept the admission of a patient who may not be a true medical case and re-route the patient once they have reached the hospital, rather than try to 'bounce' the admission whilst on the telephone to the GP. This behaviour is usually in the best interests of the patient.

When on the phone to the GP, obtain the patient's full name, date of birth and hospital number. The GP will usually write a letter which should include the patient's medication. (Prompt the GP into reminding the patient to bring the tablets to hospital.) If for any reason the GP is unable to write a letter, ask for a brief list of the patient's medication and a brief past medical history over the telephone.

Once you have accepted an admission, you should then contact the department in the hospital which will receive the patient; generally speaking this will be the ward or Casualty.

The trick to dealing with medical admissions, particularly on a busy 'take night', is to prioritise the patients. This is best done according to who needs the most urgent assessment and therapy, and this consideration should override chronological order of admission.

Priority must be given to dealing with conditions which 'will kill the patient overnight'. To help identify these, consider (for each diagnosis) 'what might happen in seconds, minutes and hours' after admission. This will also help to remind you of the priorities in the management of each medical condition.

Take the example of myocardial infarction:
- What might happen in seconds – ventricular fibrillation. Obtain an ECG immediately on a patient referred as a '?MI' and instruct the nurses to put the patient on a monitor. Put in an IV cannula and draw blood as you start taking the history. Complete a thorough clerk-in as soon as possible.
- What might happen in minutes – the patient must be appraised for thrombolysis. Discuss the ECG with your registrar and arrange other important tests such as the chest X-ray.
- What might happen in hours/days – the patient may develop a DVT, for example. Make sure you have prescribed antithrombosis prophylaxis. Double-check this on review the next morning or on the next round.

This is an example of how to prioritise your work, and can be used as a guide, in principle, for most medical emergency admissions.

Once a firm diagnosis has been made in a patient, it is easier to react to complications and/or clinical developments, as these can be predicted from your knowledge. As you become more experienced, you will start to institute therapy on your own, but always check your management decisions with your registrar as soon as possible.

Remember that a history comes from not only the patient (who may be unable to relate the events) but from relatives, witnesses of an accident or event, the GP or other involved professionals. If necessary, further details can usually be obtained by telephone from relatives, the GP or district nurse. Also, remember that the history is not just obtained at admission but often later. For example, in an emergency a full social history may not be available (patient too ill, no relatives etc.), or there may not be sufficient time. In these circumstances it is essential to find out the relevant details later. There is a world of difference between 'No history' and 'History not available'.

The same is true of examinations. In complex or unclear cases, or where the patient's condition is unstable, re-examination from time to time is fundamental to good medical practice.

Keep a record of admissions and GP calls so that patients do not get forgotten. On busy take nights you may find your patients are admitted all over the hospital. You need a brief aide-memoire of the names of patients, their whereabouts and their diagnostic categories – this is vital. Use the list to remind yourself that certain patients require review or re-testing. It is also a good idea to tape a list of admissions to the desk of the main ward for general reference.

Seeing emergency patients can be highly educational. Making decisions about patients is one of the areas in which new doctors have difficulties. This is often because patients have multiple problems. When faced with such patients it is often very helpful to construct a problem list, and then to ascribe a numerical order, putting the most significant problem at the top, working down towards those that are less seriously life-threatening, and on to the downright trivial. Often, when you have made such a list, what to do becomes obvious. If you are still not sure what to do with the patient, make a list of the possible options and then weigh up each one in turn. Always discuss even apparently simple problems with your SHO or registrar. Occasionally there is no right answer or option. However, remember that even in circumstances in which you are not going to institute therapy, a quiet word to the patients and/or their relatives may do a lot of good.

There is one caveat to instituting treatment, particularly when you are inexperienced – beware of being pushed by well-intentioned staff, patients or their relatives into starting therapy which may be counter-productive. An example of this would be the patient with respiratory failure and CO_2 retention for whom oxygen may be demanded.

Remember: You are the first line – you do not need to resolve all the problems presented to you. Discuss emergency admissions with your registrar as soon as possible and always involve a senior colleague in management decisions.

Accident & Emergency Department

You will probably spend many hours in the Accident & Emergency Department, or Casualty, and there are some useful ground rules which make life easier for everyone.

Remember that Casualty is a clearing station and that there is a constant pressure to move people through the department to the appropriate destinations. You will be able to stay on good terms with the casualty staff if you respond promptly to their requests to see a patient. You should go to the department as soon as you reasonably can, once you have been told that a patient is there waiting for you. It is quite unacceptable that patients should wait in Casualty for more than one hour after they have been referred to you, and if you feel that you cannot deal with all the patients within this time you should seek help from your SHO or registrar, from other house officers if they are available, or even from the casualty officers. Usually this will not be necessary because you will respond promptly, organise your work efficiently, and work rapidly and effectively (see the section on emergency admissions, above).

Remember that initial investigations may be much easier to obtain and review in A&E than when a patient has gone to the ward. In particular, you should make sure that the patient has a urine sample tested for sugar and protein and the presence of leucocytes and nitrites, and that this sample is saved for culture if required. You should also make sure that the patient has an ECG done, if this is appropriate, before leaving the department. You may have to do this yourself, or you may be fortunate to have an experienced casualty nurse who is prepared to do it for you.

Medical referrals in A&E are normally reviewed by your SHO or registrar. Those requiring intensive and urgent therapy, e.g. for MI or diabetic ketoacidosis, will usually be admitted urgently to an appropriate ward for investigation and treatment to commence.

Abdominal and chest X-rays should be arranged to be done during the patient's transfer from A&E to the ward, unless you have a suitable radiology service within the A&E Department. Try to establish with your registrar which patients will need abdominal films, so that all plain X-rays can be done on one visit to the Radiology Department.

Remember to take blood at the same time as you put up the drip, and do this before you take a detailed history and examine the patient.

You should only see in Casualty patients who are to be admitted. Patients who are referred for an opinion about possible discharge home should be seen by someone more senior on your firm. Record your history and examination in the hospital inpatient notes, but make a brief note on the casualty card of the diagnosis and the patient's destination, to help the casualty staff who may have to deal with anxious relatives trying to trace the patient.

Occasionally you may see a drunk, abusive or violent patient. Do not attempt to handle such a patient on your own. This is especially so if you are female, as such patients may see you as an easy target. Usually an experienced casualty nurse will be able to cope with the problem much better than you. Ill-judged attempts to match the patient's verbal or physical aggression will probably make matters worse. The best advice is to apply discretion rather than valour – others with more experience of these difficult situations may be able to calm things down.

If, by misfortune, you find yourself alone with a moribund patient and no help is available (registrar in theatre, casualty staff dealing with another patient), don't panic! Consider how best to call help. Is there anyone who might come to help? – medical or anaesthetic registrar, casualty consultant or your own consultant? If necessary press the emergency button to summon the resuscitation team.

Do not leave the patient alone unless you are sure it is safe to do so.

Remember: The basic rules of resuscitation are **ABC**. Make sure:

- that the patient has a clear **Airway**;
- that he or she is **Breathing** adequately (consider supplementary oxygen or assisted ventilation);
- that the **Circulation** is adequate (check pulse and blood pressure, and maintain cardiac output with intravenous fluids).

Theatre

Theatre lists

- Never change the order of a theatre list.
- Get it right first time and check with the operating surgeon before the list goes in.

Theatre lists must be submitted in good time. Individual theatres have different requirements, but it is reasonable to aim to have the list to theatre by lunchtime of the day before the operating sessions. Go through the order of the list with a senior colleague, either the registrar or consultant. They will usually put children, diabetics and day cases at the beginning of the list, with 'dirty' cases at the end. There may also be a tactical element to planning the list – short, non-urgent cases at the end of a list may be cancelled if an earlier major case takes longer than anticipated. Always try to get the order of the list clearly established *before* submitting it. It is confusing and potentially dangerous to make last-minute changes.

Check in the admissions book and the ward diary for any day cases, which are easily forgotten! Include all patients' details. For each patient give the full name, age, hospital number and ward. This is especially important for patients who are on a ward other than the one your consultant usually uses. Your consultant will not be pleased if he or she has to wait for a patient while the porters search for the right ward!

Do not use abbreviations on the theatre lists. The only exception is that EUA (examination under anaesthesia) may be allowed. Always stipulate the site and the side of the operation – for example: right inguinal hernia; EUA anal canal.

Be precise about the nature of the operation. Specify the approach to be used e.g. oesophagogastrectomy (laparotomy and right thoracotomy), as this helps the theatre staff to lay out the correct instruments. Also, make clear if any planned X-ray procedures require screening, so that the correct operating table will be used.

Patients who require intra-operative investigations such as cholangiography or frozen section histology should be clearly marked on the list. Inform the relevant department of the case in advance, and if possible with an estimate of when their services will be needed.

Inoculation risk cases

Patients known or suspected to be infected with hepatitis B or C or HIV are dealt with according to defined procedures, in order to minimise the risk of infection for other patients and staff. These procedures usually require the case to be the last on the list, and to be marked as 'inoculation risk' on the theatre list. Find out what procedure is followed in your hospital. (See also pages 19 and 60–1.)

Anaesthetists

The anaesthetist will usually come to see the patients pre-operatively. Nevertheless, it is courteous to inform the consultant anaesthetist of all cases on the list, with particular reference to any anaesthetic problems. If possible, contact him or her before 5 p.m. the day before the list. Consultant anaesthetists are sometimes elusive creatures, but the anaesthetic secretary can usually tell you their whereabouts, or whom to contact instead. If the consultant is not available, speak to the anaesthetic registrar booked for the list.

Consent

All patients going to theatre must sign a consent form. You must explain the operation and any likely complications, and witness their signature. Your role in obtaining consent is discussed in detail on pages 26–9. If a patient refuses to give consent, inform the surgeon as soon as possible.

Stomas

Before elective surgery that is likely to lead to the creation of an intestinal stoma (ileostomy, colostomy or urostomy), you should ensure that the patient is fully aware of the implications of this. Ask the stoma therapist to see the patient in good time, to offer advice and information, and to help choose the best site for the stoma.

Scrubbing up

Assisting in theatre is interesting and rewarding if you take part in the operation. Try to anticipate requirements and try not to get in the surgeon's way. Be particularly careful to give good retraction when the surgeon is working in a difficult area, but relax and stretch your fingers when the retraction is not required.

Ask the scrub nurse for scissors before the knot is tied, so that you are ready to cut the thread as the surgeon finishes. Learn how to tie knots and how to take off artery forceps smoothly with either hand.

You will get much more from your surgical house job if you go to theatre and assist at operations. This is the best way to understand what has happened during the operation, and may give you forewarning of postoperative complications. It may be the last opportunity in your career to see the pathology and relate it to the symptoms and signs you have elicited. Don't waste this opportunity!

Postoperative Care

One of your most important duties as a house surgeon is to care for patients after operation. *Always* see postoperative cases when they return to the ward, and examine them and their charts again before you go off duty. Ask the on-call house surgeon to check all patients who have had major surgery, and give your on-call colleague any background information that may help if problems arise.

Intravenous fluids

Most healthy adults can be prescribed fluids using a routine formula. Take specialist advice if you have to prescribe for children, the very elderly and patients in renal failure.

- 'One sweet and one sour' (use alternate bags of dextrose and saline) ... 'and always spice the sugar' (put added potassium in every bag of dextrose).
- Remember: 'One K, two Na, per kilo, per patient, per day.' (mmol/kg).
- 'Watch out for the little old lady.' (She has a low body weight, a low fluid requirement, and a low circulatory reserve.)

All major cases will come back to the ward with an intravenous infusion. It will be your responsibility to make sure that the prescription for IV fluids is written. The anaesthetist will tell you if there are any special requirements arising from the operation, but in general most patients do well with 3 litres of fluid per day, although elderly patients weighing less than 60 kg may require much less. Remember that normal minimal urine output is 0.5 ml/kg/hr or 12 ml/kg/day. Prescribe alternate bags of normal saline and 5% dextrose, and give the patient 60 mmol (6 g) of potassium per day. An alternative rule of thumb is to prescribe 1 mmol potassium and 2 mmol sodium for each kilogram body weight per day.

If there are excessive fluid losses, these will need to be replaced with an equal volume of appropriate fluid. Gastrointestinal secretions should be replaced by normal saline with added potassium, in addition to an allowance of 5% dextrose for insensible losses. For example, a case of postoperative duodenal fistula might show the following figures:

Output (last 24hr)		Replacement (next 24hr)	
Nasogastric	850 ml	Normal saline (0.9 M NaCl)	
Duodenal fistula	1770 ml	plus 40 mmol KCl/litre	
Total GI loss	2620 ml	. . .	2620 ml
Urine	1200 ml	Normal saline	1200 ml
Insensible	500–1000 ml	5% dextrose	500–1000 ml

In practice, the prescription will be for three litres normal saline plus potassium, one litre normal saline and one litre 5% dextrose. Adjustment of electrolyte infusion is based on daily measurement of plasma electrolytes, and occasionally on losses in drain fluids and urine. You will almost certainly need to discuss such a case with your registrar, who should also make an early decision about the need for parenteral nutrition.

Postoperative analgesia

- 'Most drugs come in one-dose ampoules.' So don't prescribe morphine 100 mg (= 10 ampoules!) – even if you think it's the right dose.

Most patients require opiate analgesia immediately after surgery. Traditionally this is given by intramuscular injection, on demand. Omnopon (papaveretum) 10–20 mg every four hours is usually suitable. An anti-emetic such as cyclizine (50 mg) or prochlorperazine (12.5 mg) should also be given simultaneously with the Omnopon.

Analgesia on demand means that patients suffer pain before they receive the analgesia. Many units are now using continuous intravenous infusions of opiates, patient-controlled analgesia, or epidural anaesthesia, to provide continuous postoperative pain relief. Consult a senior surgical or anaesthetic colleague before you set up or change the prescription for one of these.

On the second or third postoperative day most patients, even after major surgery, will have adequate pain relief from oral or rectally-administered analgesics. Many combinations of aspirin or paracetamol with opiates or opiate derivatives are available. Which to use will be decided by the degree of pain and by local practice in your hospital. Non-steroidal anti-inflammatory agents are also useful in reducing the need for opiates in postoperative analgesia.

Bloods

All major cases should have haemoglobin and urea and electrolytes measured on the first postoperative day. If the patient is still on IV fluids, repeat the U&E on the second and fourth days. Liver function tests need only be requested postoperatively if they were abnormal preoperatively and the operation was designed to normalise them. For example, in a patient who had obstructive jaundice due to gallstones, it would be reasonable to check the bilirubin five to seven days after surgery. It is pointless to repeat liver function tests at frequent intervals if they are deranged by hepatic metastases.

Diabetics and patients on parenteral nutrition require monitoring of blood sugar. It is kinder, if possible, to do one or two random blood sugars and four-hourly urine tests, than to prick your patient's fingers every four hours for a blood sugar test using reagent sticks.

Results

You may be fortunate to have a routine 'same day' service for blood counts and electrolytes. Don't waste your good fortune. Look at the results every night before you leave the ward and act on any abnormality. If you cannot rely on the hospital post to return the results, write 'Please phone' on the form. Check that the blood results you asked for in the morning have been phoned back by 4.30 p.m., so that you can go to the laboratory to track down the missing ones before 5 p.m., when the laboratory staff may all go home.

Radiology and Ancillary Professions

X-rays

Request all special investigations in person, form (and cap) in hand. There are two advantages to this. First, you can argue the case for an earlier date than the one you are offered, and the X-ray Department will be more inclined to help you out than if you send an anonymous form through the post. Second, you will then know the date that has been arranged when you are asked on the ward round. Successful house officers always seem to get the results the consultant wants in time for the next ward round.

Get to know the radiographers. If you are polite to them, your life will be much easier. It is a general rule that extra effort spent being pleasant to people in your first month is well repaid for the rest of your appointment.

When booking an IVU, it is useful to know the patient's urea and creatinine. The patient should be kept fasting when you go to ask for an emergency IVU. There may be special procedures in your hospital for booking ultrasound examinations, CT scans, isotope scans and arteriograms. Discover these procedures and follow them.

Gastrografin is used when checking an anastomosis for leaks, but barium is preferred for oesophageal obstruction because it is less toxic to the lungs.

Operative radiographs

Many biliary cases will need an operative cholangiogram. If your consultant is a specialist vascular surgeon you may have to book intra-operative arteriograms. Make sure you include these on the operation list, and be sure to book the investigation with the X-ray Department. A radiographer and equipment will have to come to theatre, so they appreciate some warning!

Postoperative studies

Patients who have T-tubes or percutaneous stents will require post-operative cholangiograms. Some surgeons always request contrast studies of oesophageal or rectal anastomosis in the early postoperative period. Find out your consultant's preference, and arrange the X-rays accordingly.

Endoscopy

Always take requests to Endoscopy personally. Ensure that you are clear in your own mind that there is enough time to prepare the patient (if this is necessary) and that the nurses are clear about how long patients must remain nil by mouth. Ensure that all appropriate tests are performed, e.g. clotting in jaundiced patients undergoing ERCP, and that abnormalities are corrected if necessary, e.g. vitamin K given to the patient with jaundice awaiting ERCP. Finally, if there is anything obvious which you think may affect the ability of the doctors to perform the endoscopy – for example severe chronic obstructive airways disease – then let the department know, and if necessary discuss with a senior colleague so that the endoscopist or bronchoscopist can be made aware of the situation.

Remember: When you book an investigation such as a special X-ray ... you are more likely to get it done if you *go and ask* rather than send a request.

Ancillary professions

You will find several other health care professionals on the ward. Patients may be visited by physiotherapists, occupational therapists, speech therapists, dietitians, pharmacists and stomatherapists. Get to know those of them who come to your ward. Discuss problem patients with these professionals, and try to involve them in planning management where appropriate. If you demonstrate an interest in their work and potential contribution there will be two benefits. Your patients will be cared for by more enthusiastic staff, whose morale is transmitted to the patients, and you will be able to call on your colleagues' services more easily when they are required. Particularly on the medical ward, the rehabilitation of your patients will mean that you liaise closely with such staff. Indeed, you may need to attend multidisciplinary liaison meetings with social workers, physios and OTs to plan the care and discharge of certain patients.

During your pre-registration year you will come across stomatherapists, control of infection nurses, pain care teams, palliative care specialists, breast counsellors and others offering specialist skills. These specialists can make a valuable contribution to the care of your patients.

Try to be sensitive to your patients' non-medical worries. You don't have to be able to sort these problems out, but you should be able to steer the correct people to see them; for example, social workers for financial/housing difficulties, or the chaplain for spiritual needs, and so on.

The medical secretary can be a useful ally. She will know where and when to contact your consultant (and when he or she would rather *not* be disturbed). She can make or break your reputation with the boss in a few words. So – treat her as part of the team, talk to her and help her in her job by giving her theatre lists and discharge letters in good time. You will be repaid in many small ways, which may include a tip-off about imminent consultant rage, an early warning of a patient arriving on the ward after a domiciliary visit, and uncomplaining last-minute typing, provided that this is the exception rather than the rule.

The Pharmacy, Pharmacists and Prescribing

The prescription and administration of drugs is a central part of medical management on all wards. However, all drugs are potentially poisonous and prescription errors can have serious consequences. There are a number of simple guidelines that will minimise the likelihood of errors occuring. This is an area where all doctors have to remain vigilant and careful. Remember, when prescribing, that if there is anything you are even slightly unsure of, always double-check with the British National Formulary (BNF) or ask for advice. (There should be a copy of the BNF on your ward drugs trolley.)

Your role may also encompass the preparation and administration of certain treatments, in addition to prescribing them, notably intravenous drugs and chemotherapy. As a source for help and advice in the prescription, preparation and administration of drugs, the ward pharmacist is an invaluable ally. General guidance on prescribing and how to complete a prescription can be found in the introductory section of the BNF. Read it. Always carry a copy with you to check the dosage and timing of drug administration. If you have not got a BNF, contact the hospital pharmacy as soon as possible to obtain one.

Prescribing

Hospital prescriptions are completed on standard proforma sheets, which are normally kept with the drug trolley or at the bottom of each patient's bed. When completing a prescription, print everything except your signature with a blue or black pen. In addition to being sure that you know the correct (generic) name of the drug being prescribed, its route of administration and the dosing schedule, you should ensure that the prescription sheet has the hospital location (i.e. ward) and the patient's details (i.e. complete name, date of birth and unit number), all documented in the correct spaces.

Ensure that the panel in which drug allergies and sensitivities are documented is complete. If there is any doubt over a drug allergy in a patient or if none is recorded, double-check with the patient and the case notes when you first prescribe a new drug. Ensure that you understand the layout of the prescription form and the manner in which different sections, e.g. the 'once only' prescriptions or the 'as required' prescriptions, are used. For certain controlled drugs, the dosage must be written in full in addition to being represented in numerals. Always sign a prescription and date it.

When a patient has completed a course of medication, indicate this by scoring the drug off with a clear single diagonal line. Do not obliterate the prescription, which is a record of treatment received. If a drug course is to be of limited duration, or a dose is to be missed, indicate this by scoring out the boxes at the relevant time point(s). Always inform the nursing staff of the duration of a treatment, and let them know of any changes. Rewrite a prescription rather than altering the dose on the chart, to avoid any potential confusion.

Make sure you are familiar with the arrangements for prescribing drugs to take home (TTOs) when a patient is discharged. Make clear to the patient (and a relative or carer if appropriate) the duration of each treatment, and which drugs need to be continued long term. Ensure that the GP is informed of the treatment schedule in sufficient detail to be able to prescribe appropriately for the patient in the community. Clearly document the instructions given to the patient in any correspondence with the GP. If the patient has been prescribed an unusual, complex or significantly altered drug regime, it is helpful to let the GP know by telephone to ensure that he or she is in the picture.

Prescription sheets tend to become dog-eared very quickly, particularly if there have been several changes to a patient's medication. The nursing staff may ask you to rewrite a prescription chart. This may seem an unimportant task, particularly when you are busy or at the end of a long day, but it is vital in order to minimise the possibility of prescribing mistakes and is an important part of ensuring that the ward runs smoothly.

Using your pharmacy

The pharmacy and pharmacists offer a number of important services, not least of which is advice on prescribing on a day-to-day basis. In addition, they offer drug information services and can advise you on possible complex drug interactions. There is an out-of-hours pharmacist on call in hospitals who will be able to assist you if an important enquiry arises outside of normal working hours or if an unusual drug is required which is locked away in the pharmacy. Make friends with the ward pharmacists – their help will be invaluable during your tenure as a house officer.

Reactions and interactions

Drug reactions are unfortunately an important cause of iatrogenic morbidity. The likelihood of a drug reaction occurring in an individual increases as the number of prescribed drugs increases. Always check the drug chart on ward rounds and stop any treatment that is no longer required. Refer to the BNF for its vital information on potential drug interactions, and if in any doubt ask for advice. Ensure that you are familiar with the more common side effects of the drugs you prescribe. This information is in the BNF. In the event of your patient developing an unexpected symptom or sign, always consider that a prescribed drug may be its cause. Be aware that certain prescribed drugs are dangerous in therapeutic doses in patients with renal or hepatic impairment. When prescribing for such patients always take care to check with the BNF, which also has chapters devoted to this problem.

Remember: All drugs are potential poisons. If you are unsure about a dose, schedule, route of administration or potential interaction, check with the BNF or the pharmacist. Safe prescribing requires continual vigilance.

Communication Skills

Difficult situations with patients and relatives

Patients and relatives can be awkward to handle for several reasons, but the commonest causes are anxiety and the feeling that they are being kept in the dark. This anxiety may be manifest as repeated questions, the expression of anger, complaints (against medical or nursing staff, the hospital food or administrative arrangements), or else as depression, particularly postoperatively.

Don't lose your temper with patients or relatives. Be patient. If someone complains, appears angry or upset, or is simply a nervous wreck, ask them to sit down and do so yourself. Use a gentle, low tone of voice. Ask them why they feel that way and listen to the answers. Try to explain and reassure, without getting excited. If you cannot calm them down, ask them to wait while you contact someone more senior to handle the problem. This may be your registrar or consultant or an administrator, as appropriate.

Complaints

Most complaints about hospital treatment arise from poor personal relationships between staff and patients or relatives. Honesty, patience and tact will usually avoid problems and take the steam out of heated arguments. Be polite at all times.

If a formal complaint is made against you, discuss the matter with your consultant, who will advise you as how best to answer the criticism. Do not be too discouraged if a complaint is made. All doctors receive them *occasionally*. If you have been open and honest in dealing with patients, and in explaining to them the effects and consequences of treatment and any complications, any complaint is more likely to be related to the patient rather than to yourself. However, if you receive more than one complaint during your six-month job, you should discuss the possible reasons with a senior colleague, in order to identify and correct any defect in your approach to patients.

It is always wise to keep full and honest notes of any discussion with a complaining patient or patient's family. Avoid the temptation to make witty or derogatory notes at the patient's expense, as the notes will be made available to the patient at his or her request. Remember that in any legal proceedings, the patient's lawyer will have access to the hospital notes. You may prefer to make and retain separately your own record of particularly difficult interviews, but it is generally better to make a full and factual entry in the notes (see pages 8–10 for advice on how to phrase this).

'Difficult' questions

Patients or their relatives often ask 'difficult' questions. These are often very sensible questions to which you don't know the answer. Perhaps you don't know the answer because no one knows, or perhaps you don't know the answer because of your inexperience. Admit to the patient the fact that you don't know because you have never previously encountered a similar case – it's nothing to be ashamed of. Tell them that you will ask your registrar or consultant about the problem, or arrange for a senior colleague to discuss it with the patient on the next ward round.

It cannot be said often enough that openness and honesty are essential in all dealings with patients and their relatives when you explain an operation or procedure, or when you discuss the prognosis of a serious condition, and when you answer questions arising from this discussion. Evasive answers simply increase the suspicion that something is being concealed.

Speaking to patients

In the inevitable rush to get all your chores done before some deadline, it is often tempting to forget that patients are human and to try to process them like inanimate objects.

Pause and consider what the patient must feel like on admission to your ward. They are likely to be feeling frightened and vulnerable.

Introduce yourself – even if they have been on the ward before, they might not have met you. Smile, shake hands, and try to establish eye contact. If possible, give patients some privacy by closing the curtains or using a spare room if you are to talk about personal or emotionally distressing matters. Remember that some patients are deaf; get an interpreter, if possible, for patients who don't speak English. Don't forget that communication is a two-way process – and take time to listen.

Bad news and terminal care

In discussion of prognosis, particularly in malignant disease, you should attempt to retain some hope for the patient, while still being truthful. These discussions are difficult and may best be conducted by someone more senior. Try to be present during such discussions, so that you may learn about the technique of giving bad news to a patient.

Care of patients who are terminally ill is very demanding. You will come across at least a few such patients, and if you face up to the responsibility you may find this a rewarding part of your job. The aim of management is to relieve symptoms and distress as completely as possible. The same rules apply as to all other patients: always see the patient each day (and never miss them out on ward rounds), because they are sensitive to any sign of neglect; enquire regularly about symptoms and what is troubling the patient, so that you can deal with these honestly and tactfully.

Caring for such patients may be emotionally draining for you. Everyone develops their own strategy to cope with these feelings. It may be helpful to discuss the patient and your reactions with your friends, your medical and nursing colleagues, or a member of the palliative care team. Don't be afraid that you will expose your own weakness by doing so. It is a sign of maturity to recognise difficult areas and try to deal with them.

Patients who have had palliative treatment for malignancy may welcome the support of a home care team or local hospice, even though they are not immediately 'terminal'. Discuss this possibility with your consultant first and then with the patient, before discharge from the hospital.

Medico-legal Matters

Your legal liability as a house officer is limited. Nevertheless, it is important to be aware that you have a legal duty to provide the best standard of care that is available. Much of the responsibility for clinical management will be taken by your senior colleagues, so it is important that you keep them fully informed of *any* patient who is admitted to the wards. It goes without saying that unexpected complications should be reported to a senior member of the team immediately.

Although your limited registration limits your primary legal responsibility for mishaps to the patient, you have, in common with all other hospital employees, at least four areas of legal accountability:

- to the public in criminal law,
- to the profession,
- to your employer through your contract of employment (civil courts and industrial tribunals), and
- to the patient for negligence, trespass and other civil wrongs.

The house officer's main responsibility is to maintain clear and comprehensive notes (see pages 8–10). If you do this you will earn the gratitude of your seniors if any medico-legal problems arise. Clear and accurate records of what took place, made at the time, and a record of observations to support opinions, will always assist any defence of a medico-legal claim.

Your responsibility to your patients includes making regular rounds and seeing each patient every day, and you must always go to see a patient if requested to do so by a member of the nursing staff. You cannot rely on someone else's assessment of a patient's condition, particularly if you are half asleep. The act of getting out of bed and walking into the ward often helps to clear your mind so that you can assess the patient properly.

Although the authority to institute or change treatment may be delegated to you by your senior colleagues, it is essential that you always ask yourself whether these colleagues should be informed or consulted before you embark on a new plan of management. Your registrar may not wish to be disturbed at 3 a.m. to be told about a patient with a symptomatic urinary infection whose sleep is disturbed by urinary frequency, but will almost certainly want to hear about a patient who develops a pyrexia and lower abdominal pain six days after anterior resection of the rectum. To give a patient antibiotics rather than arranging early re-operation in such a case might be construed as negligence. In general, when complications arise the operating surgeon is, if not happy, at least concerned to be informed about this as soon as possible. Most would wish to be involved in any decision to re-operate on one of their patients.

Criticism of colleagues

It is the generally accepted view that doctors should not indulge in criticism of their colleagues. Try never to express or imply criticism of another doctor or health professional when dealing with patients. The information you have at any time may be incomplete, particularly if it is related to you only by the patient. Even apparently excessive mis-management may be explained or justified by circumstances unknown to you. It is better not to discuss such matters at all with patients, but if the patient presses you for an opinion try to be non-committal. You can always say that you cannot easily comment without hearing the other side of the story.

While this may smack of the medical profession closing ranks and sticking together, you should remember that unguarded comments might support unsubstantiated criticism, and that this could then lead to unjustified litigation. The distress and damaged reputations which result from litigation, however unjustified and however firmly rejected in court, are considerable and you should do nothing to encourage this possibility. This code of practice may, after all, work to your own benefit one day!

Negligence or malpractice in a colleague

What should you do if you genuinely believe that a colleague is incompetent or dangerous? This is obviously an area for individual judgement, but the first step must always be to form your own opinion from established facts. Don't rely on gossip.

If you genuinely believe that a colleague is failing his patients in some way, do not attempt to mount a one-man crusade to expose him. Discuss your worries with your consultant, who will be better placed to assess the evidence, and who will have better knowledge of the appropriate procedures to be followed if there is a case to answer.

These remarks apply equally whether the object of your suspicion is a general practitioner, a hospital consultant or a junior colleague. In the last case you may be tempted to approach the person concerned directly. This may be appropriate if the problem is of a one-off nature, and if you can persuade the colleague to ask advice from his or her consultant. Nevertheless, you should still discuss the problem with your own consultant, who may have prior knowledge of your colleague and who may be able to take appropriate action and offer help and advice over a longer period of time than you can.

Remember that in all hospitals there exists a confidential mechanism for the investigation of allegations against medical practitioners of unfitness to practice through sickness, alcoholism or drug abuse. If you suspect that this might apply to any of your colleagues you *must* inform your consultant. These procedures are designed to protect patients and to help the doctor concerned to overcome any problems.

Above all, do not contribute to malicious rumour and do not denigrate the reputations of other people. Do not take the law into your own hands in any attempt to expose what you see as unacceptable practice by others. Although you may see things more clearly from the position of house officer than others higher up the scale, your case will rest on much stronger evidence if this can be gathered legitimately and openly, and is seen to be based on fact and not on rumour.

Always try to see the other doctor's point of view, and always believe the best of people until proved otherwise.

Cardiac Arrests

When patients collapse because their heart unexpectedly stops working in a hospital ward, this is termed a 'cardiac arrest'. The implication of the term is that a reversible event has occurred, which might respond to immediate action. To this end, each hospital has immediately available a cardiac arrest team which should be able to respond within minutes to an 'arrest call'. The team usually consists of a medical registrar, another junior physician (both concerned with diagnosis and management of the cardiac event), an anaesthetic registrar (who should supervise the airway and intubate if necessary), an experienced nurse (to draw up and, if necessary, administer drugs) and a porter (who will bring the defibrillation equipment).

If you are called as part of the arrest team, learn your role and perform it without fuss. As a house physician you will almost certainly be a member of the cardiac arrest team. Usually the house officer is expected to be responsible for establishing an intravenous line and to participate in effective cardiac massage and ventilation. Listen to the team leader (usually the medical registrar) and try to do what he or she asks, quickly and quietly. Try to use these occasions to learn from your seniors.

Occasionally you may find yourself either alone or the most senior person at a cardiac arrest. The single most important thing to do at the scene of an arrest is to institute effective cardiac massage and ventilation (checking a central pulse is a good way to ensure that the massage is effective).

Quickly check the pulse to confirm the arrest (occasionally an arrest call goes out when a patient has fainted). A precordial thump may be effective in restoring the pulse, if done within a few seconds of the arrest. Suck out the vomit, remove any ill-fitting dentures (well-fitting ones may enhance bag and mask ventilation), insert an oral airway, put on a face mask and ventilate the patient with an ambubag. Then start external cardiac massage. If you have help, get someone to massage while you ventilate. You do not need to intubate or put up an IV line before skilled help arrives.

Once the patient is being effectively massaged and ventilated you have more time to decide what to do. When someone arrives to help, ask them to continue massage and ventilation whilst you arrange the ECG electrodes and site an IV cannula and drip through which drugs can be given. You can then commence therapy on the basis of the ECG tracing. Remember that drugs in arrest trolleys generally come in one-dose ampoules. Don't be afraid of consulting a book or pictures of ECGs if you see a trace that you don't recognise on the monitor.

Finally – and this will not come easily at first – try and take a step back once the patient is effectively ventilated and massaged and make a careful and detached appraisal of the clinical picture, including information from the nursing staff about the patient's long-term prognosis and the ECG, then make carefully thought out management decisions.

On a surgical ward, cardiac arrest calls are infrequent. Predicted death in an incurable patient should *not* lead to an arrest call. Discuss these decisions in advance with the registrar or consultant.

Remember: If you are the first on the scene at a cardiac arrest:

- Airway
- Breathing
- Circulation

Aspects of Death

Unexpected deaths

These are distressing for nurses, relatives and you. Everyone copes with this differently. It is not helpful to ask the nurses such questions as 'Why didn't you call me sooner?', or to appear blasé. If the relatives are present, speak to them yourself. It is difficult, but should not be delegated. Ask a senior nurse to be present with you and to stay with the relatives after you leave, to comfort them and answer any further questions. If the relatives are not present, phone them, or ask a senior nurse to do so. This is not a job for a student nurse. It is often helpful to say that the patient's condition has deteriorated, and ask the relatives to come in, breaking the news of the death when they have arrived. It may be better not to give the whole truth over the telephone, so that the bad news can be given face-to-face and the appropriate support offered.

Certification of death

Always write the cause of death in the notes as well as certifying the fact of death. It is helpful for later analysis if the apparent cause of death is recorded at the time. It is also helpful to record whether or not this will be a coroner's case. Sign this entry legibly. These pieces of information are extremely helpful for the administrator or nursing staff who will almost certainly see the patient's relatives before you, the following day. If you are not going to fill in the death certificate, your colleague who does will appreciate your forethought in suggesting the immediate cause of death.

Post-mortem examination

Find out as soon as possible the views of your consultant on autopsy. Some consultants feel that permission for a post-mortem examination should be sought in all cases, in order to improve our understanding of the pathology. Others are more selective, in which case you should ask the consultant or your registrar, as soon as it is practical, whether an autopsy is required.

It is your job to ask the relatives for permission for a post-mortem. This should only be delegated in exceptional circumstances. It is usual to ask the relatives for their permission when they come to collect the death certificate and belongings on the day after the death. It is tactless to ask for a post-mortem in the same breath as announcing an unexpected death. Do not bargain or blackmail relatives into giving permission by threatening to withhold a certificate. If you can issue a certificate you must do so.

Your consultant will also wish to be informed *immediately* of any unexpected death, particularly in a postoperative patient. Most surgeons would prefer to have you call them at night with such news rather than discover the truth the following day on the ward. Do not wait until your boss hears the news from the patient's general practitioner, but make an effort to make contact straight away, or first thing the next day at the latest. It is also necessary to inform the patient's general practitioner by telephone as soon as possible.

Death certificates

Discuss the wording to be used on the certificate with your registrar. This will avoid distressed relatives being bounced from the Registrar (of Deaths) to the Coroner and back.

Refer to the Coroner (in Scotland to the Procurator Fiscal) all cases of accidental death, death as a direct result of operation, or if the patient failed to recover consciousness after surgery. You must also refer all deaths from unknown causes or where drug or alcohol addiction played a part. Accidental death is interpreted by some coroners to cover all cases in which a fall has occurred, including old ladies who die of broncho-pneumonia after fixation of a fractured neck or femur. In doubtful cases, contact the Coroner's Officer, who will give useful advice on which cases to refer.

Cremation forms

Patients who are to be cremated require a form certifying the cause of death and that there is no suspicion of foul play – after all, the evidence is going to be destroyed. Use the same wording that you put on the death certificate (this is another reason for recording the cause of death in the notes). Keep a record of all fees; they are subject to income tax. This includes any part of the fee which is diverted into mess funds.

Nominate a suitable registrar to sign Part C. This should be someone who was not involved in the care of the patient, and who has been fully registered for five years. You will usually be contacted by the doctor completing Part C to discuss the case; do not worry about this.

Infection Risks

Nowadays, we are all aware that surgeons and physicians may acquire potentially fatal infections from their patients. Our forebears lived and died with this risk. Hamilton Bailey lost a finger to a patient-acquired infection, and many others died from streptococcal or tuberculous infections. The advent of effective antibiotics and immunisation programmes abolished this risk and a generation has grown up in relative security.

You are in a new generation, which must accept the risk of viral infection, in addition to the bacterial diseases previously recognised. You should, of course, already have received appropriate immunisation against tuberculosis and hepatitis B. If you have not, then you should be immunised *now*. It is not too dramatic to say that your life may depend on it. In any event, your chosen career will certainly be infuenced if you contract chronic hepatitis B. After your hepatitis B immunisation, take the trouble to have your antibody level checked. If this is not known at the time of exposure to infection, you may well have to have an (extremely painful) injection of hyperimmune globulin to cover the possible failure of your immune system to develop antibodies.

Remember: It is your responsibility to get immunised against hepatitis B.

HIV infection

In the prevention of HIV and hepatitis B and C infection:
- Take care with sharp instruments and body fluids.
- Always wear gloves if contact with body fluids is likely.
- Resheathing needles is **dangerous**.
- Minimise exposure by routine precautions in all cases.
- Assume that all blood may be a source of infection.

While it is known that hepatitis B and C can be transmitted in the minute quantities of blood which are transferred on the tip of a surgical needle, the risks of transmission of HIV infection to health workers appear to be lower.

Infections acquired by hospital workers in the course of their duties appear to be related solely to the inoculation of blood or serum from hollow needles, often with a syringe still attached, or else from the contact of infected blood with large areas of excoriated or inflamed skin. The chances that you will be infected with HIV during the course of your work as a house officer are *extremely low*. You can help to reduce the risk by observing the following simple precautions:

- Always wear gloves when handling body fluid (examining infected wounds, inserting nasogastric tubes, flushing or cleaning drains, etc.).
- Always wear gloves during a cardiac arrest call, when blood certainly will be spilt indiscriminately.
- If you have an open wound on exposed skin, such as a healing cut or areas of psoriasis or dermatitis, wear gloves or apply an impermeable dressing as appropriate.
- Use vacuum tubes for blood samples, if these are available, in preference to a needle and syringe. This avoids the transfer of blood from syringe to tube.
- Avoid spilling or splashing blood. If this occurs, clear it up promptly and carefully yourself.
- Never resheathe needles – because most needlestick injuries occur during attempts to put the needle back into its sheath.
- Never put a sharp instrument or needle into a pocket or lapel of clothing. It may be forgotton and cause injury in the laundry.
- Always take a full sexual, social and drug history to identify patients at risk of infection.
- Even with low-risk patients, always apply the philosophy that prevention of inoculation is the best course.
- In the event of a needle-stick injury, immediately squeeze the area to ensure blood flow out of the wound, and wash the area with copious amounts of clear water. Following this, immediately seek the advice of Occupational Health.

Remember: Blood spreads viral diseases. Assume that all blood is infectious.

Organisation and Your Time

It is very obvious that good organisation will make a difficult and often exhausting year rather easier to cope with. For the first time since you became a medical student a degree of responsibility will rest directly with you. That means that it will no longer always be possible to leave the ward at a socially acceptable time. The time that you actually knock off will be determined by your patients, how much work there remains to be done, and how much of that work can be handed over reasonably to the on-call team (see the 'Hand-over' section, opposite). This is a feature of your professional career which will continue until you retire.

Often the cause of having to stay later than expected will be outside your control – the results of an emergency admission from clinic late in the afternoon, for example. Nonetheless, taking care to be well organised can save a considerable amount of time and stress, and properly sorting out your patients before handover (even if it delays your departure from the ward) will not only endear you to your colleagues but also make it less likely that your patients run into crises overnight.

Time management skills include the ability to:
- plan the day,
- prioritise,
- learn when to say no,
- plan ahead, and
- delegate.

However, your opportunities to do the last two of these may be limited as a house officer!

Don't put off jobs you find difficult, but try to get them completed as early as possible in the day. Use your common sense in timetabling your day's tasks, e.g. either clerk and take blood samples from patients as early as possible, or, if other commitments preclude clerking admissions, at least ensure that all important blood samples have been taken and investigations have been organised.

Try to get a reasonable amount of sleep (not easy if you have been invited to the mess party). It is usually very helpful to arrive on the ward at 8.00–8.30 a.m. to ensure any loose ends are tied up before the day starts and that the on-call team have been liaised with. It is important to double-check on what has happened to your patients overnight and to pick up (and appraise) any new admissions that are coming under your care. If you have been careful to complete blood forms the previous day, venesection can be undertaken by the phlebotomist and you can then start your day with a clean page in your notebook.

When on call, try to anticipate any problems that may arise on the ward. Tell the nurses that you will be coming round at a certain time to deal with routine matters. Encourage other members of staff to save routine jobs for your rounds and you will be bleeped less often. Beware though – if you say you are coming round, make sure that you do! Always visit the wards before you go to bed to check that there are no problems you can deal with now, to avoid being disturbed later.

Going Off Duty

Hand-over

It is vital to hand over your patients to the on-call house officer when you go off duty. Always speak to the person on call yourself, to pass on details of ill patients or those you are worried about. Try to anticipate potential problems, and leave any necessary instructions. Failure to do this is the single most important factor leading to the lower standard of care that you think your patients receive when you are not there personally to see that things are done properly. How would you feel, on your first weekend on call, if you were called to see one of your colleague's patients four days postoperatively, with a silent distended abdomen? You may well ask, 'Why on earth didn't he tell me what was going on before he swanned off to that party?'.

Make sure you tell the covering house officer about all actual and potential problems; for example, patients with septicaemia and low urine output, and that morning's patient with acute myocardial infarction, who 'looks OK now but might be worth looking at later this evening.' Speak to the house officer concerned – leaving messages leads to mistakes. If you leave written instructions, the best place is in the patient's notes. Good hand-over is particularly important at the weekend, when your patients will be looked after for forty-eight hours or more by doctors who are not familiar with their recent progress and who may not know the particular requirements of your consultant.

Careful hand-over takes time, but it is essential. The ideal is for both you and the covering house officer to briefly walk round the ward and comment on every patient. If your firm has a clear resuscitation policy relating to a patient, ensure that it is handed over to the on-call staff and understood by the nursing staff.

Remember: 'Leaving messages leads to mistakes.' Always convey important information, and hand over details of patients, directly to the person concerned.

On-call rota

It is the collective responsibility of the house officers to make their on-call rota work. As with annual leave, it is important that you and your colleagues coordinate your activities. Check that the rota is accurate, and correct any mistakes and inconsistencies. If you think a better rota could be devised, work it out with your colleagues and present it to the consultants. In general, medical staffing officers do not understand the rotas and will be delighted to accept your version.

Annual leave

Take your annual leave. It is an entitlement and not a privilege, and if you don't take it no one will notice. Arrange with the other house officers that you will not all be away at the same time, and tell your consultant, registrar and Medical Staffing of your holiday plans in good time. It is also helpful to inform the medical secretary and switchboard. Last-minute arrangements are no good, because time is needed to arrange locum cover.

Sickness

Don't be foolish. If you are ill, stay off work, and if necessary see your GP. You are less efficient, and may infect your patients. Despite all rumours to the contrary, you are not indispensable (but remember that too much time off will prevent you being signed up for registration!).

Your Contract

Your contract is very important. It is a legally binding document that protects both you and your employer. You must therefore read your contract very carefully and understand it before you sign it. Do this *before* you start work. Contracts follow a nationally agreed model, and should include the following points:

- Your contracted commitments in terms of hours of duty.
- Your pattern of work in terms of the on-call rota or shifts.
- Your salary.
- Your leave entitlement.
- The requirement for you to be resident.
- The date on which you take up and finish employment.
- The notice of termination that you are to give or entitled to receive.
- A clause that prohibits the employing authority from making deductions from or variations to your salary without your expressed written consent.
- Limitations on your obligation to perform unpaid duties.

One part of each contract is the job description. This is supposed to give you information describing the job in such a way that you can gain a reasonable and accurate picture of the living and working conditions, as well as the full duties of the post and the training that it offers. In the UK you can get further information on contracts and job descriptions from the series of leaflets published by the British Medical Association. If there is a problem with your contract or if you do not receive your contract, or if it does not conform to the nationally agreed model, the BMA suggest that you contact them. If you have a more trivial worry about your contract it is often a good idea to speak to the incumbent house officer before you start, to check that you would be working on the same basis. Remember that once you sign a contract it is legally binding on both parties.

At the time of writing it was accepted that individual Trust hospitals in the UK would continue to adhere to the nationally agreed terms of employment and nationally agreed contract models. Obviously this may change in the future.

Medical Indemnity

Since 1990, hospital doctors in the UK have been indemnified by their NHS employing authorities. This means that any claim for negligence arising as a result of your work in the hospital is effectively insured against by your employer. However, the British Medical Association and the Department of Health both strongly advise all doctors to take out defence body membership or some form of personal indemnity insurance to cover situations outside the hospital, such as 'good Samaritan' intervention and private practice.

How to Make Sure You Are Getting Trained

The Pre-Registration House Officer year is designed as a formal part of your medical education. This is why you are not eligible for full registration with the General Medical Council until you have completed the Pre-Registration year. During this time the Regional Postgraduate Dean is responsible for ensuring that your training is adequate, and will have nominated one consultant to be your educational supervisor during each six-month post.

The first step in making sure you are getting adequate training is to identify your educational supervisor, and to check your weekly programme with him or her. Your educational supervisor is not necessarily the consultant you are working with when you start the post, particularly if you rotate between different firms. The job of the educational supervisor is to review your progress at least twice during your post, so that deficiencies in your training can be remedied and your overall progress can be assessed.

However, it is most important that you realise that this process is your responsibility. The onus is on you to complete your training record and to discuss it with the educational supervisor. It is up to you to identify deficiencies in your training programme and make these known, so that they can then be remedied. Various institutions and mechanisms exist to help you get a good training and some of these are discussed in detail below.

Remember: The educational value of the post will be improved if constructive criticism is received from you.

Induction day

Each six-month house officer post in the UK should begin with an induction day. It is essential that you attend this because you will be given useful information about local practice in your hospital. You will be given a mountain of paperwork which you should take time to go through, because each piece of paper has a specific function. Unless you have read the hospital major incident plan, for example, you will not be able to find your way through it in an emergency. You may find it helpful to use the space provided at the end of this book to make a record of local protocols discussed during the induction day.

The induction day will be in protected time – that is, you will not be expected to answer clinical commitments during that time. Arrangements will be made for someone else to carry your bleep. Hand it over and do not feel guilty. Most contracts now specify a full day induction for those starting in August and a half day induction for those starting in February. Don't miss it!

Formal teaching

Check your weekly programme to see when there are formal teaching sessions. These may take the shape of postgraduate training time for all junior staff, there may be special lectures or seminars dedicated to education for house officers, and there will be activities on your own firm or department which involve house officer education. Examples of these include case presentations, audit meetings with review of complicated cases, and grand rounds. Pathology and X-ray meetings will serve to give you background information about the investigation and diagnosis of the patients under your care, and are often highly educational.

Do not be tempted to skip these meetings to get your clinical work done. They are an important part of the pre-registration year and should take precedence over all but life-threatening emergencies. Find out if there is a system in place for dealing with bleeps and phone calls during this teaching time. For example, if there is a specific time for house officer teaching, will your SHO carry your bleep? If the whole directorate is attending an afternoon training session, is there one person designated to answer all bleeps, etc? Are the nurses on the ward aware that you are in a teaching or educational session, so that they can save all non-urgent calls until your return to the ward?

A useful way to encourage the ward to retain non-urgent requests until you are on the ward, rather than bleep you, is to have a message board with dry marker pens so that any requests for replacement IV lines, prescriptions for analgesia, etc. can be written up until you are able to deal with them. This system will only work if you respond to the messages regularly and in a timely way.

Ward rounds

Postgraduate training is essentially an apprenticeship system, despite the great improvements that have been made in formal teaching over the last few years. You should take every opportunity to profit from the experience of your seniors. Discuss patients on ward rounds so that any questions you do not understand can be answered on the spot. Do not be afraid to ask questions about any aspect of the patient's care. Informal discussion of difficult cases or recurrent problems can take place at any time, with your registrar over lunch, for example, and your consultant will probably be delighted to explain why he or she chooses a particular approach to the conditions in an area of special interest – you should take every opportunity to find out why things are done in a particular way on your firm.

A useful educational resource neglected by some house surgeons is the opportunity to assist in the operating theatre. Not only does this give you an excellent demonstration of living pathology, but it is also an opportunity to begin to acquire surgical skills if you are interested in a surgical career. Perhaps the greatest educational benefit of operating, however, is the time spent in enforced conversation with your consultant or registrar. This will let you explore difficult areas, ask for clarification, and even get some career advice from a variety of people.

The same opportunities do not generally exist on medical firms. Nevertheless, you should seize every opportunity to undertake practical procedures such as insertion of central lines, joint aspiration/ injections and so on. If you have the opportunity to attend GI endoscopy lists, ERCP or bronchoscopies etc., do so. Your colleagues will usually welcome a spare set of hands. In addition, even if you seek a career in general practice, having a good working knowledge of what these procedures entail will enable you to advise and support your future patients.

Educational record

The Postgraduate Dean (through the Postgraduate Clinical Tutor) will give you an educational record book which will contain a proforma method of self-assessment and joint assessment with your educational supervisor. Use this record to assess your own training after two months in the post. Discuss with your educational supervisor the good and bad points of the training you receive, and identify any areas which require attention. Your educational supervisor will go over the progress you have made so far, and together you will agree areas to be addressed over the next three months. This conversation must take place in 'protected time', so you should give your bleep to a colleague.

You should repeat this process after five months in post to review the progress that has been made. The educational record is your property and your responsibility. It is a very powerful tool to improve the education that you receive during the job, as well as to modify practice for your successors. Use it!

Get into the habit of using the review process as a framework to analyse your strengths and difficulties. You will then be able to apply it throughout your career. This will help you to become a better medical practitioner.

How to get help and resolve problems

If you feel that your educational needs are being ignored, there are several people who can help you. Initially you should discuss the problem with those who can most easily rectify it. If, for example, your consultant appears too busy to answer questions or explain management during a ward round, ask if there is a suitable time when you could discuss difficult patients. If there is no formal educational activity timetable, discuss with your registrar when it could be fitted in, and jointly approach the consultant with a plan of how to establish it.

If you feel unable to approach your consultant, or if you do so without success, the next person to go to is the College Tutor for Medicine or Surgery, as appropriate, or the Postgraduate Clinical Tutor. They will be able to offer advice about timetables of educational activities, and ways in which you can increase your exposure. A clinical tutor will no doubt be able to point to a formal educational programme in the Postgraduate Centre, so you should go prepared with an explanation as to why that is insufficient, and what are your specific educational needs that can be rectified by additional activities.

If all of these avenues fail to produce an improvement, approach the Postgraduate Dean directly. The Postgraduate Dean is a joint University and NHS appointment, and has responsibility for supervision of all postgraduate training in addition to house officers. The Dean is Chairman of the Regional Pre-Registration House Officer Committee, which has a very influential role in the organisation and approval of house officer posts. Do not underestimate the Dean's power. If he or she requires change in your timetable it must be complied with. You are most likely to get a positive response and support if you can demonstrate that you have already attempted to resolve the problem locally and that despite these attempts a serious educational deficit still exists. You can obtain the Dean's address from the secretary or administrator in the Postgraduate Centre of your hospital.

Your own responsibility

In addition to attending the formal educational programme, you should set aside time for private study. Use this time to read current journals in your speciality, to find out more about interesting or difficult cases. The habit that you should have developed as a student, of reading about the conditions of the patients you have clerked, should now be ingrained, but you will necessarily become more focused on the unusual and interesting cases. This method of reading around your clinical experience is a painless way to acquire knowledge and improve your understanding. The link with clinical experience helps to fix the reading clearly in your memory.

You are responsible for ensuring that your educational programme is adequate, and for discussing your progress with your educational supervisor.

Remember: The house officer year is part of your training. Take every opportunity to pursue formal and informal educational activity.

How to Obtain Counselling and Career Advice

We approach this topic with some hesitation. It is a brave wedding guest who proffers his services to the happy couple as a marriage guidance counsellor! Nevertheless it is true that being a house officer is a stressful occupation, and there is no shame in recognising when the stress is sufficiently great for you to seek advice and help. Furthermore, counselling covers areas of career advice and overlaps with the provision of training, which you are advised elsewhere in this book to pursue actively.

Who needs counselling?

Nearly all doctors in training seek advice and help at some stage. The times when you are particularly likely to benefit from counselling are:

- when you try to decide your next career step;
- when you want to know how to apply for your next post;
- when you are faced with an emotionally difficult or draining clinical situation;
- when you have to deal with aggressive relatives, violent behaviour or aggrieved patients;
- when you find that personal antagonism with other members of staff is affecting your work.

There are several other chapters in this book which offer advice for many of these difficulties. This chapter tells you in broad terms where to go to discuss particular problems.

Informal counselling

Traditionally, junior hospital doctors have developed a 'sufferers' support network' which functions, like many admirable patient support networks, to provide help and advice through the grapevine of shared experience and understanding. Or to put it more simply, the best person to ask about how to survive the miseries of house jobs may be your SHO.

Career planning

It is not too soon or too late to plan the next few years of your career. First you must decide what broad area you wish to work in, and if you have no clear intention already, try to talk to as many different specialist trainees as possible during your pre-registration year.

Don't forget that there are many other interesting and challenging occupations for a doctor outside of general practice and the major clinical specialities in the hospital. Public health medicine, medical research in a university, medical responsibility for product development in the pharmaceutical industry and medical journalism are some of the alternatives you could consider. Your local Director of Public Health or the Medical Director of a drug company will probably be delighted to explain the attractions and rewards of their job.

However, you will also need to consider how to make the next step on your journey to an SHO post. Someone who has recently done that, such as your present SHO, is well placed to advise you. Don't restrict yourself to the SHO on your own team, but discuss career options and approaches to job applications with all of your colleagues in the training grades. (See also page 79.)

Dealing with stress

If you are fortunate you will have had some instruction in stress management as an undergraduate. Your own personal strategy is important. Try to recognise priorities in your work and order your day appropriately. Accept that your power to influence some clinical or administrative problems may be limited. Do your best, but recognise that failure to achieve a perfect result may be due to factors outside your control. The next level of stress management involves recognising that stress exists, and then talking about it either informally or formally with colleagues and counsellers.

It is often helpful to get right away from work when you are off duty. If you have an opportunity to live outside the hospital, perhaps in a flat or house with friends, think seriously about taking it. Physically leaving the hospital is a good way to unwind. Taking regular exercise, for example swimming, can also be very therapeutic. As already mentioned, take your annual leave.

If you are uncertain how to handle a difficult clinical problem, or how to deal with awkward interpersonal relationships, it may be helpful to discuss it with your colleagues who may be experiencing similar difficulties. Even simply airing the problem and recognising that other people are also suffering the same problem can be a tremendous moral support. It is surprising how often discussing a problem can make its resolution obvious.

The people you spend most time with are likely to be the senior nursing staff on the wards. There is often an opportunity for quiet discussion over a cup of coffee while relaxing on an evening shift, or during the quieter moments of the day. A recently qualified staff nurse may not have sufficient experience to recognise your own difficulties, but those with more experience, whether they are senior staff nurses, ward managers or nurse managers, may well be able to give you some friendly advice or a sympathetic ear. Who to talk to is a matter of personal choice and personalities.

Before you unburden yourself, ask yourself whether the person you are talking to is someone you can trust to give you sensible advice and to be discreet.

Talk to your consultant

Your consultant is likely to be concerned about your welfare and interested in you personally. Most consultants recognise that happy house officers generally perform better than those who have become disgruntled or disillusioned. It is therefore in their interest to help resolve any difficulties you may have. Furthermore, most of them have benefited from the informal network described above and are only too happy to contribute their own advice and opinions to those you have gathered from junior colleagues.

For house surgeons, the opportunity to discuss problems may arise in theatre or in the relative privacy of the surgeons' room or changing area. House physicians may have similar opportunities during the boss's cardiac catheter or endoscopy lists, and it is surprising how often you can raise specific problems and get specific advice during the course of the weekly routine of ward rounds, or outpatients, and while waiting for formal teaching sessions to start. It is also always possible to arrange an interview in your consultant's office. Whatever course you adopt, you do however have to take the initiative – your consultant has many things on his or her mind, and while happy to respond, may not enquire very frequently about your own state of mind.

Formal counselling

If you feel that you are suffering unduly from stress or that you are receiving inadequate training in important areas of the job, to the detriment of your own mental wellbeing, you should urgently approach one of the people with responsibility for your welfare:

Your educational supervisor (who may not be your current consultant);
The clinical tutor in your speciality (medicine or surgery);
The postgraduate tutor in the hospital;
The Postgraduate Dean.

All of these should respond rapidly to a request for help, and if you feel desperate you should make a request personally by telephone. If you believe you will have difficulty with one of these individuals, or feel that one is inappropriate (perhaps because of personal difficulties), then do not hesitate to contact one of the others.

In an ideal set-up you will have regular and frequent contacts with at least two of the people on the above list, and these should be approached first. However, if no such contacts exist, do not hesitate to beat a path to the door of the most accessible of them, as they will undoubtedly respond positively in urgent circumstances.

Remember: It is better to talk than to suffer in silence. You will deal with stress more positively if you attempt to catch up on sleep, eat regular meals and don't over-indulge in alcohol.

How to Write a CV and Apply for an SHO Post

You may already have prepared a curriculum vitae in your applications for your house officer post, although many medical schools operate computer matching schemes which do not require a CV. In any case, your CV will need revision in order to make it suitable for application at the next level.

At this stage your CV will seem fairly short, and even with appropriate spacing and balancing the layout it is unlikely to run to more than two sides of A4. You will need to amend your CV regularly to include all your most recent experience, as potential employers are much more interested in your experiences since qualification than in the details of your pre-clinical or school education. However, when applying for your first SHO post you should start with your A-level results and any other significant achievements at school, and work forwards from there.

There is a fairly conventional layout for a CV, and following it will help a prospective employer to look through the information you present and quickly find what he or she is looking for. When drafting your CV, you should use a good word-processing package, and choose a variety of fonts and typefaces to give the overall presentation a clean and clear appearance. Make full use of headings.

The following outline gives a fairly standard pattern for constructing a CV, and you should try to find something to include under as many headings as possible. Show the completed draft to your boss – and his secretary! They will both be used to sifting through piles of CVs and will be able to advise you and offer constructive criticism (and the secretary may offer to re-process the final version!).

OUTLINE FOR A CURRICULUM VITAE

Personal details
Name

Date of birth

Marital status and children – if relevant. These are customary but may be omitted, if you prefer.

Address. Include a reliable postal address and your work address. A reliable daytime telephone (and fax) number is invaluable for the personnel officer.

GMC registration number and date of full registration

MDU/MPS/MDDUS membership number

Present employment
Give a reliable telephone number and fax number where you can be contacted during working hours, for example your boss's secretary. Give the names of the consultants you work for, the hospital, and the grade of your present post.

Employment history
List in chronological order the posts you have held since qualification. Do not include short locums, but any locum appointment longer than one week is probably worth including at this stage in your career, particularly if you gained exposure to a speciality you have not worked in elsewhere. For each post, list the consultants with whom you have worked and their particular interests.

List any relevant employment before starting your medical course and any employment during vacations, etc. For example, if you worked as a laboratory technician between school and university, include that. Mention any work in a hospital as an undergraduate, e.g. nursing auxiliary, porter, etc. Do not include employment as barman in the Students' Union.

Education
This should be divided into three sections: school, undergraduate and postgraduate. Under each heading include significant examination results, starting with A-levels and include any grades, honours or distinctions. Under postgraduate education you should include any teaching activity or courses you have attended.

You should list any courses or conferences attended and state the purpose, and what you gained from the course. If you have completed a project or similar piece of work at any stage in your career, describe it briefly and state what you learned or achieved as a result.

Prizes and Awards

You should make specific mention of any undergraduate or other prizes you have won for academic achievements. List separately any awards or fellowships you have won (for travel during your elective period, for example), and any official fellowships or scholarships gained during your training.

Postgraduate experience

This section should be a descriptive paragraph or two outlining the experience you have gained in the different posts you have worked in so far. In this section you can point out any special expertise you have gained, and emphasise the skills you have acquired along the way.

Postgraduate qualifications and diplomas

If you are still in your pre-registration year it is unlikely that you will have sat any postgraduate examinations. This section will become relevant when you have passed one of the Primary or Part I examinations of one of the Royal Colleges, for example.

Publications

It is unlikely that you will have had the opportunity to undertake research projects and present the findings. Nonetheless, if you have done so, any presentations and publications, be they abstracts, case reports or full research papers, should be given prominence on your CV.

Do not worry if you have none yet, but remember that in many fields publication is taken as evidence of enthusiasm and application. Look out for opportunities to publish case reports, or to take part in research projects.

Hobbies and interests

This section is optional. It is often thought to be superfluous, but we believe it to be important because it gives you an opportunity to include any special distinguishing features. For example, if you play golf or tennis at county standard this may be of interest to a potential employer. Moreover, being captain of a team or secretary of a club usually demonstrates organisational or simple managerial experience which a future employer may look on favourably.

How to apply for the post

Writing the CV is only the first step in applying for an SHO post. The next step is to decide what kind of post you want, and where it will lead you to. Many house officers find that the next logical step is a six-month Casualty post. This has two definite advantages. It allows a period of training in which greater responsibility will be given to you to make decisions and institute treatment. This is a very 'character building' experience, and properly supervised it is invaluable. The other advantage of a Casualty post is that it is often a very good entry into a hospital in which you wish to work on an SHO rotation. This gives you a referee within the hospital, and allows you to meet other junior staff and find out about possible future vacancies. It enables you to attend postgraduate meetings in your chosen speciality, and makes sure that the local consultants know who you are.

If you wish to enter a medical/surgical rotation or vocational training scheme, ask as many colleagues as possible about available rotations. When you have decided where the next post is going to lead you, you should look for the appropriate immediate and long-term combinations. Having identified a suitable post, make sure you are ahead of the game. Keep an eye on the BMJ classified section from about the fourth month of your *first* post, so that you get a feel for what may be available six months later. If you see an attractive rotation which will start before you are fully registered, it may be to your advantage to ask the consultant in charge for more information and for an estimate of when the next vacancy will arise.

Many SHO posts attract large numbers of applicants, and some consultants prefer to make appointments without advertisement. This is possible for one-off posts, but is increasingly not the case with posts within rotations. Nevertheless, you will do yourself no harm by approaching the consultants for whom you wish to work, introducing yourself and indicating your interest in their post. At this stage it is helpful to inform your current boss of your interest and of any contacts you make. Then if your boss meets the target consultant, a few informal words of support will reinforce the good impression you have already made. If this is not possible, a polite request that your boss telephones the target consultant can be invaluable.

It is beyond the scope of this book to describe how to improve interview skills, but you should aim to do so for career interviews and examination vivas. Several books exist (see the Reading List).

Educational Assessment of First Post

Name of educational supervisor:

Date of 1st assessment:

Outcome of 1st assessment:

Plan for change:

Date of 2nd assessment:

Outcome of 2nd assessment and remedial action if required:

Date of final assessment:

Outcome of final assessment:

Educational Assessment of Second Post

Name of educational supervisor:

Date of 1st assessment:

Outcome of 1st assessment:

Plan for change:

Date of 2nd assessment:

Outcome of 2nd assessment and remedial action if required:

Date of final assessment:

Outcome of final assessment:

Checklists

These lists are appropriate to the start of either your house surgeon or house physician post. They will also be useful if you rotate to a different firm during your appointment.

Before you start

You should contact your predecessor well in advance (remember that the final two weeks are a favourite time for holidays). You should find out:

- What is the timetable? (in as much detail as possible)
- When will be my first night on call?
- Does the consultant have any particular prejudices or preferences in treatment, for example, *never* use gentamicin, *always* use prophylactic heparin?
- What is the best way to contact anaesthetists for routine lists (telephone numbers and best times to call)?
- Who is the most approachable member of (a) the surgical/medical team, and (b) the nursing staff, to help sort out problems in the first few days? (But beware of relying too heavily on someone else's assessments of character – make your own judgements!)
- Which services in the hospital are helpful, and which services are difficult to deal with or need careful handling?
- Which radiologist and pathologist is best to approach with urgent problems?
- What is the routine for out-of-hours and Saturday morning blood tests?
- What days do the routine admissions come in on?
- Any tips for ensuring that day cases are seen and sorted out quickly?
- Are there any specialist pathologists/radiologists that your firm liaises with?
- Is there a pre-admission clinic?
- Where is the doctors' mess, and is it habitable?
- Can we meet to hand over the patients on the day before I start?
- Failing this, where will you leave a list of explanatory notes on each patient?

Important things to do and ask on your first day

There should be an induction session for new house officers. You must attend this if it is available. You will be told about all hospital routines, from how to use the telephone to how to manage a cardiac arrest. (Take this book along, and fill in or modify the checklists.)

If you don't know the hospital, establish the geography as soon as possible. You need to know your way to:

- All the surgical or medical wards (on your first night on call you don't want to get lost)
- A&E Department
- Theatres
- Radiology Department
- Pathology labs
- Canteen
- Doctors' mess
- Medical staffing office
- Telephone exchange

Things to ask the registrar

- Check the timetable with the registrar.
- Check the on-call rota.
- Ask about routines for preoperative investigation, investigations before interventional procedure, prophylactic antibiotics and pro-phylactic heparin.
- Is there a routine plan for dealing with the common emergencies (e.g., the SHO appraises all ?MI cases)?
- Run over your duties and role on the firm.
- What bloods does the firm obtain in common emergencies?
- Are there established protocols for the intake of patients (e.g. upper GI bleeds go to physicians, lower GI bleeds go to surgeons)?
- Who takes the admission calls?
- What are the arrangements for handing back patients previously under another firm?
- Is there a cross-matching policy?
- Can I ring you at home when you are off duty if one of our patients develops a problem? If so, what is your home telephone number?

More general things to do

- Introduce yourself to the nurses on all the medical or surgical wards, and in theatres or the Endoscopy unit if appropriate, and in the A&E Department.
- Find your consultant as soon as possible and remind him of your name, giving him as much information as possible in your first breath, so that he can appear to remember all about you. ('Hello Mr Knife. I'm Jenny Willing, your new house surgeon. I've just done my finals at . . . / I've just finished my medical house job with Dr Goode at . . . ').
- Visit Medical Staffing to sign contracts and to present your Registration Certificate.
- See all your patients.
- Check the progress of investigations and arrange new ones according to your registrar's instructions.
- Put in tomorrow's theatre list (see pages 37, 87) and telephone the anaesthetist.
- Write out the routine investigations (bloods, X-rays and ECGs) for the next morning.
- Try to meet your fellow house officers at the end of the day to unwind and compare notes.
- Congratulate yourself on surviving so far.

Finally, *read* all the circulars, information, protocols and handouts you have been given. *Some* will contain invaluable advice. Make notes of important items in the blank pages at the back of this book, and amend other parts to record local practice.

Before the patient is discharged from the ward

- Has the patient (and/or relatives) made adequate arrangements for care at home? You may need to ask the relatives and/or the nursing staff.
- Does the patient understand his or her part in rehabilitation (e.g. exercise after an MI)?
- Does the patient need to go to a convalescence hospital or nursing home before finally going home? (This may take several days to arrange – think ahead.)

- Does the patient need any medication to take home?
  - Continue pre-existing treatment.
  - Explain any new treatment carefully to the patient.
  - Ensure the patient knows the duration of treatment.
  - Explain possible side effects and give advice on driving and alcohol consumption.
  - Tell the patient what to do if a dose is forgotten. (Don't worry; Take the next dose as planned; Take a dose as soon as you realise.)
- What follow-up arrangements should be made?
  - When and where should the patient come to Outpatients?
  - Does the district nurse need to call?
  - Does the patient need to visit his/her GP?
  - When should any sutures be removed?
  - Who should remove them?
- Does the patient have a discharge letter to take to the GP?
- Have you seen all relevant investigations and histology reports? If these are outstanding, keep a note of the patient's name, and remember to find the results.

Summary of preoperative investigations

- Always investigate appropriately any symptom.
- Patients who take diuretics need U&E.
- Patients who take anti-hypertensives need ECG.
- Asian patients need CXR (?TB).
- Afro-Caribbean patients need a sickle test.
- History of jaundice – hepatitis screen.
- High alcohol intake – prothrombin time.
- In the case of an otherwise fit patient for elective surgery, only do the following:

Over age 40	Full blood count
Over age 50	Full blood count + ECG
Over age 60	Full blood count + ECG + U&E + CXR

- For medical/interventional radiology procedures, see pages 43–4.

How to prepare for a ward round

- Check all the patients and know which wards they are on.
- Routine admissions:
  - Outpatient and GP investigations done and results available?
  - All X-rays present?
  - Any new findings since clinic?
  - Any problems that might affect plans for surgery or programmed investigations?
- Unresolved problems:
  - Summarise present status.
  - All blood results up-to-date?
  - Recent investigations available?
- Are there any ward referrals?
- Is the theatre/endoscopy/procedure list clear, or are the details available for the consultant to plan it?

When a patient dies

The nurse in charge of the ward will inform you and ask you to see the patient. Do this as soon as possible, because the body may not be moved until certified dead.
- Verify the fact of death.
- Record in the notes:
  - Evidence on which you conclude that the patient is dead.
  - Date and time of death and of your examination.
  - Cause of death as it appears to you, and whether the coroner should be informed.
- *If the relatives are present.* Speak to the relatives and answer their questions. Make sure someone offers them a cup of tea.
- *If the relatives are absent.* Make contact by telephone (yourself or a senior nurse). Explain the circumstances or ask relatives to attend as appropriate. Ask the relatives to come the next day for administrative reasons.
- *Next day.* Issue death certificate or inform the Coroner (Procurator Fiscal in Scotland). Request post-mortem examination, and answer relatives' questions.

How to book an emergency case with theatre

- Decision to operate confirmed by registrar.
- Inform theatre. Give the nurse in charge full details: diagnosis, operation, patient's name, date of birth, hospital or A&E number, ward and operating surgeon. *And* – find out when a theatre will be available.
- If the patient is still in the A&E Department, arrange a bed on the ward, and either admit to ward, or arrange admission *via* theatre.
- Contact anaesthetist with all clinical details and information as for theatre (above). Agree a provisional operating time. Ask if any pre-medication is needed.
- Inform other interested parties, such as ward nurse, radiographer.
- Confirm time with theatre. Send patient to theatre or ward as appropriate.
- Check that all blood results, X-rays, ECG, cross-matched blood are available before patient goes to theatre and that the patient has signed a consent form.

Theatre lists

For each patient you need to know: Name, Age, Ward, Operation: name – site – side.

- Confirm the order of the list with the operating surgeon.
- Take the list to the secretary or theatre in time.
- Patients who need cross-match:
  – Serum sent.
  – Blood available in theatre fridge.
- Inform anaesthetist of patients on list (the previous day if possible).
- Make sure that all relevant investigations are available (e.g. U&E, CXR, ECG).
- Is the consent form signed and the operative site marked in each case?
- Inform ancillary services:
  – Frozen section.
  – Operative radiography.

Medical/interventional radiology procedures

- All require consent.
- *Renal biopsy.* Up-to-date IVP, urine and blood, creatinine, protein and electrolytes, full blood count, clotting, group and save, MSU, IV cannula. If any results are deranged, discuss with registrar.
- *Cardiac catheter.* ECG, chest X-ray PA and lateral, FBC, fasting cholesterol, clotting, group and save, patient nil by mouth, IV cannula. If any results are deranged, discuss with registrar.
- *Bronchoscopy.* Chest X-ray PA and lateral, pulmonary function tests, arterial blood gases, ECG, patient nil by mouth, may require IV cannula. If any results are deranged, discuss with registrar.
- *Liver biopsy/Injection of varices.* Clotting, FBC for platelets, group and save, IV cannula sited. If any results are deranged, discuss immediately with registrar.
- *ERCP.* Clotting, full blood count, site IV cannula, patient nil by mouth. Correct clotting with vitamin K if indicated. If any results are deranged, discuss with registrar.

NORMAL VALUES

Most laboratories report the normal range alongside the patient's results. Use your own laboratory's reference range rather than published figures. Below are some common values, in case of need.

HB	12–15g/dl
WBC	3–10.5 $\times$ 10^6/l
Platelets	100–950 $\times$ 10^9/l
Sodium	130–148 mmol/l
Potassium	3.3–4.6 mmol/l
Bicarbonate	19–30 mmol/l
Urea	3–7 mmol/l
Creatinine	<90 μmol/l
Bilirubin	<17 μmol/l
Alkaline phosphatase	90–330 u/l
Albumin	35–42 g/l
AST	<40 u/l
Calcium	2.2–2.6 mmol/l
Blood glucose (fasting)	3.6–5.4 mmol/l
Amylase	70–300 u/100 ml

Correct calcium values for low albumin: to the observed value, add 0.02 x (40–Alb).

ANTHROPOMETRIC FIGURES

Patients rarely know their body weight in kilograms. Surgeons and anaesthetists no longer work in the Stone Age. Always convert the patient to standard medical (i.e. metric) weights and heights:

stones	kg	ft.	ins.	cm	stones	kg	ft.	ins.	cm
1	6.4	5	0	152	12	76.4	5	9	175
2	12.7	5	1	155	13	82.7	5	10	178
5	31.8	5	2	157	14	89.1	5	11	180
6	38.2	5	3	160	15	95.5	6	0	183
7	44.5	5	4	163	16	101.8	6	1	185
8	50.9	5	5	165	17	108.2	6	2	188
9	57.3	5	6	168	18	114.5	6	3	190
10	63.6	5	7	170	19	120.9	6	4	193
11	70.0	5	8	173	20	127.2			

Postscript

We hope these pieces of advice will help you get through the year ahead of you. At times your job will seem intolerable. The rewards of job satisfaction, grateful patients and intellectual stimulation may seem very distant at 2 a.m. as you work through your eighteenth admission of the day and your bleep goes yet again to call you to theatre, or to the ward to write up night sedation, or to answer yet another call from the GP deputising service. At times like these you will feel that being a house officer is rather like growing mushrooms (they keep you in the dark and every so often someone opens the door and shovels more manure on your head). Remember, though, that mushrooms grow quickly, and in a few short months you will have finished your house jobs and you will become an SHO, perhaps with a house officer of your own. Like your present SHO, you will be knowledgeable, quick thinking, calm in a crisis, and always ready with an addition to the poor house officer's differential diagnosis. Perhaps you then will be able to pass on some of the advice in this book, and quite probably you will have some additions from your own experience.

Keep your head down and keep going. The first priority is to survive the bad patches and enjoy the good patches to the full.

Looking through this book we see that it is essentially about communication. The house officer is the focal point through which all the information relating to the patients on the ward should flow.

Remember:
- Ask for advice when necessary.
- Tell everything you know about the patient.
- Talk honestly to patients and on equal terms to other members of the team.

Suggested Additional Reading

Duties of a Doctor, 1995. Guidance from the General Medical Council.

Fisken, R. A., 1994. *House Physician's Survival Guide*. Churchill Livingstone.

Hill, G. and Farndon, J. R., 1994. *Guide for House Surgeons and Interns in the Surgical Unit* (9th edn). Butterworth-Heinemann.

Hope, R. D., Longmore, J. M., Hodgetts, T. J. and Ramrakata, P. S., 1994. *Oxford Handbook of Clinical Medicine* (3rd edn). Oxford University Press.

McKee, R. F. and Scott, E. M., 1987. 'The value of routine pre-operative investigations.' *Ann. Roy. Coll. Surg.*: **69**, 160–2.

Roberts, C., 1985. *The Interview Game and How It's Played*. BBC Books.

Robinson, R. and Stott, R., 1993. *Medical Emergencies – Diagnosis and Management* (6th edn). Butterworth-Heinemann.

Saunders, M., 1987. 'Problems with notes.' *J. Med. Defence Union:* **3**, 10–11.

'Surgery and long-term medication.' *Drug Ther. Bull.* 1984: **22**, 73–6.

Local Protocols

The headings on the following twelve pages can be used to record local practice.

MAJOR INCIDENT PLAN

Record here your responsibilities should there be a major incident. You will find details of this in the hospital major incident plan. It is your employer's responsibility to ensure that you receive a copy of this when you take up your appointment.

Action if on duty:

Action if at work but not on call:

Action if off duty:

ROUTINE ANTIBIOTIC PROPHYLAXIS

ANTICOAGULATION PROTOCOL/DVT PROPHYLAXIS

SLIDING SCALE FOR INSULIN THERAPY/ PERIOPERATIVE INSULIN REGIME

IMMEDIATE CARE OF MYOCARDIAL INFARCTION

IMMEDIATE CARE OF CRESCENDO ANGINA

IMMEDIATE CARE OF ACUTE ASTHMA

IMMEDIATE CARE OF COAD EXACERBATION

IMMEDIATE CARE OF PULMONARY EMBOLUS

IMMEDIATE CARE OF GASTROINTESTINAL BLEEDING

IMMEDIATE CARE OF DIABETIC KETOACIDOSIS

IMMEDIATE CARE OF OVERDOSES

Tricyclic antidepressants:

Paracetamol:

Salicylates:

Phone Numbers

INTERNAL PHONE AND BLEEP NUMBERS

Wards: _____

_____

_____

_____

_____

ITU: _____

Theatre: _____

A&E sister: _____

A&E doctor's office: _____

Administration office: _____

Outpatients appointments: _____

OP consultant's room: _____

OP registrar's room: _____

Consultant's office: _____

Consultant's secretary: _____

Registrar/Senior reg.: _____

SHO: _____

Other HO: _____

_____

_____

_____

Medical registrar: _____

_____

Surgical registrar: _____

_____

Doctors' mess: _____

_____

Clinical services manager: _____

_____

Unit bed manager: _____

Haematology results: _____

– emergency requests: _____

Biochemistry results: _____

– emergency requests: _____

Blood bank: _____

Microbiology results: _____

– emergency requests: _____

Histology reception: _____

– results: _____

– frozen section: _____

Cytology: _____

X-ray Department: _____

– routine: _____

– portables: _____

– bariums: _____

CT: _____

Ultrasound: _____

Nuclear medicine/imaging: _____

Other: _____

On-call radiographer: _____

Physiotherapist: _____

Dietitian: _____

Social worker: _____

Pharmacy: _____

Porters: _____

Medical Illustration: _____

'Patients' office' (death certificates): _____

Medical Staffing office: _____

OUTSIDE PHONE NUMBERS

Check whether your hospital switchboard has tie lines or abbreviated codes for any of these numbers.

SHO (home): _____   _____

Registrar/Senior reg. (home): _____   _____

Consultant (home): _____   _____

– private secretary: _____   _____

Consultant anaesthetist (home): ____   _____

_____   _____

_____   _____

Coroner: _____   _____

Local hospitals (NHS and private): ___   _____

_____   _____

_____   _____

_____   _____

_____   _____

_____   _____

_____   _____

Large local general practices/health centres or GPs who send a lot of patients to your consultant:

_____   _____

_____   _____

_____   _____

_____   _____

_____   _____

_____   _____

_____   _____

_____   _____

INDEX

Booklets for Patients from Beaconsfield Publishers

Hysterectomy and Vaginal Repair, Sally Haslett, RGN, RHV, RM and Molly Jennings MCSP, 28pp, 3rd edn 1992, ISBN 0906584310

Explains the meaning and effect of these operations and describes how to prepare for them. Advice on what to do afterwards for a trouble-free return to normal life.

'*This booklet has proved its worth over and over again.*'   Woman's Realm

Having Gynaecological Surgery, Sally Haslett, RGN, RHV, RM and Molly Jennings MCSP, 30pp, 1995, ISBN 0986584396

Parallel booklet with the above, with advice on preparation for and recovery from gynaecological surgery other than hysterectomy or vaginal repair.

'*I would recommend this booklet to anyone who is about to embark on gynaecological surgery.*'   Physiotherapy

Having a Cervical Smear, Sally Haslett, RGN, RHV, RM, 21pp, 1994, ISBN 0906584388

Answers questions by women. Describes the test, the different investigations and treatments, and explains the technical terms a doctor or nurse might use.

'*In a clear, sympathetic and readable style, Sally Haslett has anticipated fully all the possible fears and anxieties associated with cervical cytology.*'   Brit. J. Sexual Medicine

Lymphoedema: Advice on Treatment, Dr Claud Regnard, Caroline Badger RGN and Dr Peter Mortimer, 24pp, 2nd edn 1991, ISBN 0906584329

Explains what the condition is, and provides a daily management plan that can be followed at home.

'*This little booklet is a model of a guide to self-help.*'   Patient Voice

Oral Morphine: Information for Patients, Families and Friends, Dr Robert Twycross and Dr Sylvia Lack, 24pp, 1988, ISBN 0906584221

Brings together answers to questions frequently asked by patients.

'*Answers many of the questions raised by patients and families when morphine is introduced in the treatment of cancer pain.*'
Palliative Medicine

The Early Days of Grieving, Revd Derek Nuttall, 26pp, 1991, ISBN 0906584299

Offers support, explanation and information, speaking directly to the bereaved person.

'*The author does this without becoming sentimental, mawkish or doctrinaire.*'   The Lancet